Researching Complementary and Alternative Medicine

Complementary and alternative medicine (CAM) has become big business around the world. Alongside the growing consumption and provision of CAM has emerged a small but growing body of research exploring the area. Nevertheless, research on this topic is still in its infancy and there is a real and urgent need to investigate CAM further.

Researching Complementary and Alternative Medicine brings together leading researchers from Australia, Canada, Germany, New Zealand, Norway, the UK and the USA, and constitutes a valuable and timely resource for those looking to understand, initiate and expand the investigation of CAM. Contributors draw upon their own CAM research work and experience to explain and review a range of methods and research issues pertinent to the contemporary field of CAM and its future development, such as:

- the issues facing practitioners who wish to conduct research;
- how and why qualitative methods should be used alongside quantitative methods;
- how the randomised-control trial method relates to CAM;
- the potential of developing consumer involvement in research;
- the challenges of conducting CAM systematic reviews.

This book will be essential reading for students and academics in CAM, health studies, health social science and public health. The book will also be relevant reading for medical students and CAM, medical and other health-care professionals.

Jon Adams is Senior Lecturer at the School of Population Health, University of Queensland and Visiting Research Fellow at the School of Healthcare Studies, University of Leeds, UK. Jon has researched and published extensively on aspects of CAM and he is Associate Editor for the journal *Complementary Therapies in Medicine*.

Contents

Illustrations

Figures

Tables

Notes on contributors

Jon Adams is a Senior Lecturer in Social Science Related to Health at the School of Population Health, University of Queensland, Australia. He is also a Visiting Research Fellow at the University of Leeds, UK and is Associate Editor of the journal *Complementary Therapies in Medicine*. His research interests include the consumption, practice and provision of CAM in Australia and Europe and the interface between CAM and general practice, nursing and midwifery.

David Aldridge is the Chair for Qualitative Research in Medicine in the Faculty of Medicine, Universität Witten Herdecke, Germany and is Honorary Visiting Professor for Creative Arts Therapies in the Department of Health Care at the University of Bradford, UK. He specialises in developing research methods suitable for various therapeutic initiatives, including the creative arts therapies, complementary medicine and nursing. He teaches and supervises research in medicine, music therapy, the creative arts and nursing.

Penelope Carroll is completing her Ph.D. in the Department of Public Health, Wellington School of Medicine and Health Sciences. A CAM practitioner, journalist and researcher, her writing and research focuses on issues of power and social justice with an interest in presenting the validity of alternative and often competing perspectives.

Marc Cohen is the Founding Professor of Complementary Medicine at Royal Melbourne Institute of Technology University, Australia and the President of the Australasian Integrative Medicine Association. He plays an active role in both researching and teaching CAM and is the past Founding Director of the Centre for Complementary Medicine at the Monash Institute for Health Services Research at Monash University, Australia.

Kevin Dew is a Senior Lecturer in the Department of Public Health, Wellington School of Medicine and Health Sciences, New Zealand. He has research interests in many fields including CAM, health inequalities and aspects of health communication and interaction. A linking thread in his various research interests is the legitimation of knowledge claims in health.

Jeanette Ezzo is Director of Research at JPS Enterprises, Baltimore, Md., USA. She is the past Cochrane Complementary Medicine Field Administrator and the past Systematic Reviews Co-ordinator in the Division of Complementary Medicine, University of Maryland Medical School. She has published systematic reviews on acupuncture, massage and mind–body therapies.

Eric Manheimer has worked with the Cochrane Collaboration since 1997, and he has been involved with the preparation of multiple systematic reviews of CAM therapies. He currently serves as the Administrator of the CAM Field of the Cochrane Collaboration and the Director of Database and Evaluation at the Center for Integrative Medicine, University of Maryland School of Medicine, USA.

Charlotte Paterson is an experienced general practitioner and a Medical Research Council special training fellow in health services research at the University of Bristol, UK. Her ten-year research programme has combined qualitative and quantitative methods and has focused on patient perspectives of acupuncture and how to define and measure patient-centred outcomes.

Marie Pirotta is an experienced general practitioner and a Senior Lecturer at the Department of General Practice, University of Melbourne, Australia. Her research interests are in women's health, CAM and randomised controlled trials. She also teaches clinical skills and general practice in the undergraduate medical programme.

David Sibbritt is a Senior Lecturer in Biostatistics at the Centre for Clinical Epidemiology and Biostatistics, University of Newcastle, Australia. He is an experienced biostatistician with a variety of health research interests, including CAM. He is also the Statistical Advisor to the journal *Complementary Therapies in Medicine*.

Aslak Steinsbekk is a Research Fellow at the Department of Public Health and General Practice, Norwegian University of Science and Technology, Norway. He is currently researching patient education and user involvement. He previously worked as a homoeopath in private practice for twelve years and has undertaken epidemiological research, qualitative research and randomised controlled trials in CAM.

Laura C. Vanderheyden is a Ph.D. candidate at the Department of Community Health Sciences, University of Calgary, Canada. Her research interests are in CAM and the meaning and use of different types of evidence in patient decision-making.

Marja J. Verhoef is a Professor in the Department of Community Health Sciences at the University of Calgary, Canada. She holds a Canadian Research Chair in Complementary Medicine. Her research interests include developing appropriate methodological approaches to evaluate complementary and alternative therapies and examining factors related to patient decision-making.

Acknowledgements

I am grateful to *Annals of Internal Medicine* for permission to reproduce Figure 2 in Chapter 2.

Abbreviations

CAM	complementary and alternative medicine
DSI	daily stress inventory
EBM	evidence-based medicine
GEE	general estimating equations
GP	general practitioner
IBS	irritable bowel syndrome
MAR	missing at random
MBSR	mindfulness-based stress reduction
MCAR	missing completely at random
MHF	Mental Health Foundation
MHI	mental health index
MLD	manual lymphatic drainage
MMR	measles-mumps-rubella
MNAR	missing not at random
NHIS	National Health Interview Survey
NCCAM	National Center for Complementary and Alternative Medicine (USA)
NHL	Norske Homeopaters Landsforbund (Norwegian Homoeopathic Society)
NHS	National Health Service (UK)
NRC	Norwegian Research Council
NSAIDs	non-steroidal anti-inflammatory drugs
PBS	Pharmaceuticals benefit schedule
QALY	quality adjusted life year
RCT	randomised controlled trial
SDA	secondary data analysis
SSRI	selective serotonin reuptake inhibitors
TCM	traditional Chinese medicine
WHO	World Health Organisation

Introduction

Jon Adams

The rise of complementary and alternative medicine (CAM) – a whole array of practices, products and approaches to health and illness[1] – can certainly no longer be characterised as cultural fad or fashion. Changes in the use of titles (from 'unscientific' and 'marginal' to 'complementary' and 'integrative') reflect a more substantive relocation and transformation of many of these medicines from the fringe to the mainstream of both community and professional health-care discourse and practice (Tovey et al. 2004). The most recent reports from various late modern societies suggest the use of CAM is a widespread phenomenon amongst patient groups (Girgis et al. 2005) and the general public (Adams et al. 2003, Barnes et al. 2004), and one which is being allocated extensive out-of-pocket personal funding (MacLennan et al. 2002, MacLennan et al. 2006).

Quite apart from the ever-expanding range of self-care products and technologies, CAM is increasingly found in the solo or group practices of therapists working predominantly outside the state-sponsored health system. Yet, CAM practice is not confined to the swelling ranks of private therapists but is also beginning to make its presence felt in more conventional areas of health-care delivery such as general practice, nursing, midwifery and even the more traditionally conservative conclaves of certain hospital specialisms (Samano et al. 2005). The numbers of those within such lines of practice and who are now recruits or supporters of CAM have, in some cases, reached a relatively significant proportion, and professional representative bodies are increasingly taking note of the 'dissenters' or 'entrepreneurs' (depending upon their point of view) within their ranks (BMA 2000, RCNA 1997). Indeed, CAM has fast become identified as a pressing public health issue (Bodeker and Kronenberg 2002, Giordano et al. 2003) with implications for health-care practice, provision and the equity of and access to care. Such implications have not been lost on governments (House of Lords 2000, Expert Committee on Complementary Medicine in the Health System 2003).

Given these developments, it is not surprising that CAM is finally shaking off its status as a topic beyond the research gaze. Despite the fact that CAM research activity remains relatively small-scale when compared to the resources allocated to conventional health research, the past couple of decades have seen the emergence of a number of peer-reviewed journals dedicated to CAM (e.g. *Complementary Therapies in Medicine* and *Journal of Alternative and Complementary Medicine*) and the medicines are now beginning to occupy the interest of a growing number of investigators (Bensoussan and Lewith 2004, Fontanarosa 2001). University CAM departments have also emerged (with particular pockets of concentrated activity in Australia, Canada, the UK and the USA) (Hentschel 2002); funding programmes and organisations dedicated to investigating and promoting an understanding of CAM are now well established (e.g. the Research Council for Complementary Medicine, UK and the National Center for Complementary and Alternative Medicine, National Institutes of Health, US); and an International Society for Complementary Medicine Research (ISCMR) has recently been founded (Lewith and Verhoef 2006).

The move towards integrative medicine (whereby CAM and conventional treatments find ever closer relationship in clinical care) has fuelled the drive to assess the efficacy of different CAM therapeutics. This is undoubtedly a worthwhile pursuit made ever more pressing by the need for health-care systems to effectively allocate limited resources. As a number of chapters in this collection attest, we are still moving towards refining instruments and gathering the evidence from such inquiry.

However, there is a danger of tying the CAM research programme exclusively to the issue of efficacy. In order to fully understand CAM we must broaden our approach beyond simply asking questions of clinical effectiveness, to include methods and research perspectives from neighbouring traditions such as public health, health-services research and health social science. This broadening of scope does not belittle the role and significance of clinical research and the search for a clinical evidence base for CAM. On the contrary, a multidisciplinary, multi-method approach supports and strengthens such clinical research, providing a wider context for understanding practice, developing reflection and shaping sensitive policies and directives in the field of CAM.

Fortunately, the contemporary research enterprise around CAM is now undoubtedly swelling with interest from an ever broadening cast of disciplines and groupings. As health research more generally has embraced multidisciplinary collaboration and teamwork, so too has the evolving field of CAM inquiry. Despite the occasional dissenting voice pressing for the exclusion of important methods and approaches (Ernst 2005), it is widely supported that a range and mix of methods and paradigms is desirable, indeed essential, if we are to address the far-reaching research questions posed by CAM and its recent ascendance. Such a broad model of investigation is to be applauded and provides the backdrop for the collection presented here.

To date, most books in the CAM field have followed a somewhat restricted agenda concerning themselves with either: the investigations of one group or grouping of perspectives (for example the social sciences [Tovey et al. 2004], legal issues [Stone and Matthews 1996] or a clinical focus [Ernst 2001, Lewith et al. 2002]); or the professional development of clinicians through the provision of 'how to' CAM guidebooks (Cross 2000, Yates 2003). However, as this collection illustrates, there exists a larger pool of investigators who are utilising a wide range of approaches and methods and who are engaged in exploring and understanding CAM. This book provides the first wide-ranging collection of methods and issues selected from across the 'broad church' that can be identified as the CAM research community.

Book outline and contents

The aim of *Researching Complementary and Alternative Medicine* is to draw together wide-ranging pieces focusing upon various aspects of the research enterprise to help inform and advance the investigation and understanding of CAM. The explosion of interest in these medicines as a worthy research topic is essentially international in scope, and in response the collection brings together contributors from Australia, Canada, Germany, New Zealand, Norway, the UK and the USA. Authors have also been purposefully selected for their spread of disciplinary groundings and expertise including biostatistics, public-health research, health social science, general practice and CAM therapy amongst others.

All contributing authors are active CAM researchers and all draw upon their own research agendas and experiences, and that of others in their area, in order to highlight and discuss key issues and challenges from the field. While authors may employ case studies based upon an individual therapy or set of therapies/practices, the – aim wherever possible – is focused upon providing insight and discussion of relevance to those engaged or interested in any of a wide range of CAM.

The attempt to investigate and examine CAM (in terms of a broad research movement) is plainly an enormous endeavour and is ultimately beyond the scope of any one collection. There are topics and methods grounded in other disciplinary approaches (for example, economics, history and pharmacology) that currently provide valuable contributions to the exploration and investigation of CAM yet are not included in this book. No apology is made for such omissions, restricted as this book is by space and resources, save to explain that such topics and methods are not purposefully neglected nor undervalued. This book does not aim to be exhaustive nor comprehensive in its coverage but instead presents a number of topics that have been identified as significant by a selection of leading researchers grounded in the grass roots of empirical CAM inquiry.

This book is divided into two parts: 'Methods in Practice' and 'Issues from the Field'. While the topics presented are distinct they do often interrelate and overlap in practice, and it is hoped that readers will certainly turn to a number of chapters in the book in line with not only their immediate interests and requirements but also a curiosity and desire to develop and enhance their reading or research adventures.

Part I, 'Methods in Practice' explores a selection of methods as a means of investigating CAM. One area often overlooked but attracting attention of late is the use of qualitative research and methods to explore CAM, a trend signalling the growing interest in this topic of health and health care from within the social and behavioural sciences. Qualitative methods can play an important role in combined-methods design (as we will see later in this collection). However, qualitative inquiry of CAM does not necessarily have to be employed alongside or supplementary to more traditional approaches to health research. In recognition of this fact, and in an attempt to help dispel the idea that this approach to research is an afterthought or inferior to other types of inquiry, this collection opens with discussion of qualitative research and methods in relation to CAM.

In Chapter 1, Aldridge explores the potential role for a narrative approach and aspects of the accompanying qualitative perspective in the investigation of CAM. As Aldridge highlights, with a focus upon the practices of spiritual healing and prayer, the interpretative framework can be extremely useful for examining the ways in which we tell our stories of falling ill and becoming well. This is a framework that sits comfortably with the need for a multiple perspective to CAM research that does not start and end with a positivist approach.

Moving to what will be for many perhaps more familiar territory (at least for those engaged in or trained in clinical practice and research), Chapter 2 explores the method of systematic reviews for examining CAM. As Manheimer and Ezzo identify, there has been an explosion in the number of systematic reviews of CAM over the past two decades or so. However, in addition to the methodological issues that face all reviews, CAM systematic reviewers have to address additional challenges given the complexity of CAM interventions. Manheimer and Ezzo illustrate, through case studies of their own work and that of others in the field, various approaches used to address some core methodological difficulties facing those looking to consider or conduct meta-analysis with regard to CAM.

A secondary analysis is not confined to systematic reviews, and in Chapter 3 Sibbritt draws upon his own work to outline the potential contribution of analysing existing large cohort study data to investigate CAM use and CAM users. Despite some particular difficulties – often the consequence of design decisions taken prior to the CAM researchers' involvement in the study – Sibbritt explains how utilising existing data sets, where possible, can have some attractive benefits for the well-positioned researcher or research team seeking to examine CAM consumption.

Returning from a population health to a clinical focus, Pirotta (Chapter 4) explores the application of the randomised controlled trial (RCT) method for

CAM. As she explains, the development of the RCT for CAM is at a critical stage – one characterised by great opportunities and serious methodological challenges. Pirotta explores a number of developments in RCT design that have attempted to overcome some of the core problems in the field and she suggests there are reasons to remain optimistic that further progress can be achieved in the application of RCT method to the study of CAM.

In line with a multi-method, multi-perspective approach and closing Part I of the collection, Verhoef and Vanderheyden describe how qualitative and quantitative designs (RCT) – two approaches that are perceived by some as incommensurable – can be combined to examine CAM interventions. Verhoef and Vanderheyden outline the argument for such a methodological integration and the movement towards CAM whole systems research as well as charting some of the barriers to combining qualitative research approaches and RCTs. While whole systems research is still in its relative infancy and, as the authors rightly explain, there remains a need for further conceptual and operational groundwork, this emerging field holds much promise for advancing the investigation of CAM interventions.

Developing multidisciplinary, multi-perspective research in CAM quite obviously necessitates an engagement with methods of many sorts. However, perhaps a less striking implication of such a broad multifaceted approach to CAM research is the introduction of a critical reflection upon the fundamental ideals, concepts and processes of the wider CAM research experience. As such, in Part II the collection redirects attention away from specific designs and methods to contemplate a selection of significant issues currently occupying a number of investigators in the field. Identifying and developing an evidence base for practice is a growing movement within contemporary health care (McLaughlin 2001) and the consequences of such a movement for CAM appear mixed (Willis and White 2004). The second part of the book opens with an argument by Cohen (Chapter 6) that while evidence is certainly the cornerstone to developing a rigorous scientific approach to CAM, collecting and interpreting evidence is not necessarily the same for CAM as it is for more conventional treatments. He explores a number of key issues around the production and appropriation of evidence for CAM with reference to treatment decision-making as well as the broader political and social context.

One criticism, often aimed primarily at clinical CAM research but also relevant to associated investigations, is that study aims, designs and findings are sometimes removed, if not divorced, from the requirements of clinical practice and the concerns of practitioners. It is essential to acknowledge that not all research should be moulded around a policy or practice agenda (this would be to deny the full contribution of critical analyses such as that offered by social science) (Tovey et al. 2004).

Nevertheless, the relationship between research and practice is a concern that needs to be addressed if we are serious about improving patient care and health. Some have proposed a central role for practitioners in researching their own CAM as a means of grounding the research agenda in practice realities. This is a suggestion that not only suits a multidisciplinary team approach but also promotes utilising the services of those within the growing ranks of CAM therapy – an otherwise untapped resource for research production. As Steinsbekk (Chapter 7) explains, programmes in a number of countries have attempted to promote the idea of practitioner as researcher. Drawing upon his experience of one such programme, he highlights various hurdles, both at the individual and broader therapy level, with regard to research capacity-building from within CAM practice.

In Chapter 8, Dew and Carroll explore the relationship between CAM and public health. As we saw in Chapter 3, traditional perspectives and methods of population health inquiry can help illuminate aspects of CAM consumption. However, Dew and Carroll ask more fundamental questions of public health employing CAM and related perspectives to probe and reflect upon the frameworks and assumptions of public health as a discipline. As their analysis of the frameworks used by traditional public health and those associated directly or indirectly with CAM highlights, the relationship between the two fields is often contrasting and problematic.

To close the collection, Paterson explores the role and involvement of consumers in CAM research. In a similar vein to encouraging practitioners' participation in conducting research, this final chapter outlines the possible benefits of inviting consumers to become resourceful members of the research team. The bulk of CAM research (not unlike health research more generally) has employed and perpetuated the model of researcher as 'expert' and the consumer as 'non-expert'. Yet, as Paterson explains, the consumer perspective is important and useful at all stages of the research process and, if encouraged and harnessed carefully, may prove a highly significant resource for a marginalised field such as CAM.

While a multi-method, multi-perspective approach is an ideal goal for CAM research, it is not without its challenges and difficulties. A quick search of the research literature and editorials/think pieces cannot fail to identify the controversy and debate within the field (for example, see Vickers 1999). The same as CAM practice is not a homogenous world (housing a vast range of practices and practitioners), so too does division and subdivision permeate the conceptualisation of a CAM research community. This is not a weakness of the CAM domain but the stuff of *all* scientific fields of inquiry (Cozzens and Gieryn 1990).

Moreover, highlighting debate is a necessary and healthy requirement of any establishing field. As such, it is hoped that this collection will act as a springboard for many readers helping to introduce what, for them, may be new methods and issues and ultimately producing CAM inquiry grounded in critical self-reflection and an openness to other paradigms rather than a dogmatic entrenchment along disciplinary boundary lines.

Importantly, it is envisaged that the collection will also have wider appeal and readership than simply those with an interest or engagement in the substantive topic of CAM. To disregard CAM research activity is to overlook a potentially rich source of innovation for all health researchers. Research methods along with issues such as the role and context of evidence, the role of the practitioner as researcher and the promotion of consumer involvement in the research process are of relevance and significance to the wider field of health research. CAM, with its status of the 'other' and its often presented paradigm clash with conventional care and the biomedical model (Coulter 2004) provides an excellent case study for constructively questioning, reevaluating and refining the application of established tools and approaches to broader health research.

Note

1 The inclusion of specific therapies and treatments under the heading of complementary and alternative medicine is temporally and spatially variable. However, while remaining mindful of such variability, CAM here refers to those healing practices, technologies, perspectives and products (within a given country and at a given time) that are not an established component of conventional medicine.

References

Adams, J., Sibbritt, D., Easthope, G. and Young, A. (2003) 'The profile of women who consult alternative health practitioners in Australia', *Medical Journal of Australia*, 179 (6): 297–300.

Barnes, P., Powell-Griner, E., McFann, K. and Nahin, R. L. (2004) 'Complementary and alternative medicine use among adults: United States, 2002', *Advance Data*, 27 (343): 1–19.

Bensoussan, A. and Lewith, G. T. (2004) 'Complementary medicine research in Australia: a strategy for the future', *Medical Journal of Australia*, 181 (6): 331–3.

Bodeker, G. and Kronenberg, F. (2002) 'A public health agenda for traditional, complementary, and alternative medicine', *American Journal of Public Health*, 92 (10): 1592–1.

British Medical Association (2000) *Acupuncture: Efficacy, Safety and Practice*, London: BMA.

Coulter, I. (2004) 'Integration and paradigm clash: the practical difficulties of integrative medicine', in P. Tovey, G. Easthope and J. Adams (eds) *The Mainstreaming of Complementary and Alternative Medicine: Studies in Social Context*, London: Routledge, pp. 103–22.

Cozzens, S. E. and Gieryn, T. F. (eds) (1990) *Theories of Science in Society*, Bloomington, Ind.: Indiana University Press.

Cross, J. (2000) *Acupressure: Clinical Application in Musculoskeletal Conditions*, Oxford: Butterworth Heinemann.

Ernst, E. (ed.) (2001) *The Desktop Guide to Complementary and Alternative Medicine: An Evidence-Based Approach*, Edinburgh: Mosby.

—— (2005) 'Keynote comment: dumbing down of complementary medicine', *Lancet Oncology*, 6 (7): 442–3.

Expert Committee on Complementary Medicines in the Health System (2003) *Complementary Medicines in the Australian Health System: Report to Parliament Secretary to the Minister for Health and Ageing*, Canberra: The Committee.

Fontanarosa, P. B. (2001) 'Publication of complementary and alternative medicine research in mainstream biomedical journals', *Journal of Alternative and Complementary Medicine*, 7 (1): 139–43.

Giordano, J., Garcia, M. K., Boatwright, D. and Klein, K. (2003) 'Complementary and alternative medicine in mainstream public health: a role for research in fostering integration', *Journal of Alternative and Complementary Medicine*, 9 (3): 441–5.

Girgis, A., Adams, J. and Sibbritt, D. (2005) 'The use of complementary and alternative therapies by patients with cancer', *Oncology Research*, 15 (15): 281–9.

Hentschel, C. (2002) 'Profiling "centres of excellence" in CAM research', *Complementary Therapies in Medicine*, 10: 46–8.

House of Lords (2000) *Complementary and Alternative Medicine*, London: House of Lords.

Lewith, G. T., Jonas, W. B. and Walach, H. (eds) (2002) *Clinical Research in Complementary Therapies: Principles, Problems and Solutions*, Edinburgh: Churchill Livingstone.

Lewith, G. T. and Verhoef, M. J. (2006) 'The international society for complementary medicine research (ISCMR): the way forward', *eCAM* (doi:10.1093/ecam/nek004).

McLaughlin, J. (2001) 'EBM and risk: rhetorical resources in the articulation of professional identity', *Journal of Management in Medicine*, 15 (4–5): 352–63.

MacLennan, A. H., Wilson, D. H. and Taylor, A. W. (2002) 'The escalating cost and prevalence of alternative medicine', *Preventive Medicine*, 35: 166–73.

MacLennan, A. H., Myers, S. P. and Taylor, A. W. (2006) 'The continuing use of complementary and alternative medicine in South Australia: costs and beliefs in 2004', *Medical Journal of Australia*, 184 (1): 27–31.

Royal College of Nursing Australia (1997) *Complementary Therapies in Australian Nursing Practice: Position Statement*, Canberra: RCNA.

Samano, E. S., Ribeiro, L. M., Campos, A. S., Lewin, F., Filho, E. S., Goldenstein, P. T., Costa, L. J. and del Giglio, A. (2005) 'Use of complementary and alternative medicine by Brazilian oncologists', *European Journal of Cancer Care*, 14 (2): 143–8.

Stone, J. and Matthews, J. (1996) *Complementary Medicine and the Law*, Oxford: Clarendon Press.

Tovey, P., Easthope, G. and Adams, J. (eds) (2004) *The Mainstreaming of Complementary and Alternative Medicine: Studies in Social Context*, London: Routledge.

Vickers, A. (1999) 'Reflections on complementary medicine research in the UK', *Complementary Therapies in Medicine*, 7 (4): 199–200.

Willis, E. and White, K. (2004) 'Evidence-based medicine and CAM', in P. Tovey, G. Easthope and J. Adams (eds) *The Mainstreaming of Complementary and Alternative Medicine: Studies in Social Context*, London: Routledge, pp. 49–63.

Yates, S. (2003) *Shiatsu for Midwives*, New York: Books for Midwives.

Part I

Methods in practice

Chapter 1

Qualitative methods in CAM research

A focus upon narratives, prayer and spiritual healing

David Aldridge

Introduction

The daily life of a researcher and research supervisor is helping people make sense of what they do. Life is literally about making sense, with the activity on making – this is a constructivist approach to human knowledge that fits well with the broad spectrum of methods known as qualitative research (Denzin and Lincoln 1994). When we talk about what we do, this also includes health and sickness talk. We talk about falling ill and becoming well. How we regain health, and what that status of health is, is reflected in the ways in which we talk about it and how we explain this to others.

When we recall how sickness fell upon us and how we regained our health then we inevitably tell a story; these are the narrative approaches to life that we have. Narratives have characters, events and themes, and these are the very stuff of qualitative research (Williams et al. 2005). One of the difficulties of medical research is that while being increasingly proficient at refining concepts of disease and their treatment, there is little headway being made into those areas where health is defined and how that seemingly elusive status that we know as health can be achieved.

In response to such circumstances, this chapter explores the role of a narrative approach and aspects of the accompanying qualitative perspective necessary to help investigate and understand dimensions of health and CAM. To illustrate this qualitative research perspective, the chapter focuses upon the practices of spiritual healing and prayer, areas where the advantages of a qualitative approach can be clearly identified.

Qualitative research and definitions of health

Health care is invariably defined in positivist terms as an object, phenomenon or a delivery system (Aldridge 2004a). Knowledge gained through scientific and experimental research is deemed objective, quantifiable, stable and measurable (at best measurable by instrumentation reducing human error). In qualitative approaches, however, we have a shift in paradigm. Knowledge about health is considered to be a process, a lived experience, interpretative, changing and subjective (at best gleaned through human interaction as personal relationship). Indeed, from this qualitative perspective we may be encouraged to think of the gerund form of the word 'health' as 'healthing'. In the same way, we can also consider what we do as professionals, and what our patients are involved in continually, as the relationship of healing (Aldridge 2000, Aldridge 2004a, Aldridge 2004b).

Qualitative research is not a testing mode of inquiry but a discerning form of inquiry requiring the collaborative involvement of those participating in that healing relationship. This emphasis on the verb 'healing' rather than on the noun 'health' goes some way to explain why qualitative approaches have found such resonance in *nursing* research, with its emphasis on *nursing* and *caring* as relational activities, rather than *health-care* research, which is by definition nominal and objective.

If healing is a relationship, then we have to ask ourselves how we evaluate relationships. Would we take friendship, for example, and rate it on a one to five Likert scale or would we value our friendships for their various qualities? It is possible to meaningfully explain to another person what the value of a relationship is without quantifying it if we wish to demonstrate the nature of that friendship. So too for the relationship that is healing. We need to discern those personal qualities that people use to explain healing. However, this is a major opposition between scientific paradigms and the first question often asked of qualitative research in medicine is, 'Is it scientific?' The short reply to which is, 'Yes, it is social science'.

Medicine, being a social activity, is susceptible to being understood by a social-science paradigm as much as it is by a natural-science paradigm (Mechanic 1968, Kleinman 1973). To fulfil the functions of health-caring adequately, we need both quantitative and qualitative approaches. While medical science may concentrate on the external laws of the universe, qualitative research will concentrate on our internal understandings and their coherence with the way in which we live our lives.

Social psychology, ethnography and medical anthropology are acceptable scientific approaches for studying human behaviour, and qualitative research takes much of its methods from those fields. Indeed, suffering, distress, pain and death are experiences relevant to understanding health care but elusive to measurement. Similarly, well-being, hope, faith, living a full life and satisfaction are experiences central to health care but not immediately amenable to quantification. But they can be apprehended by understanding (Lewinsohn 1998) and these understandings are gleaned in relationship, the central activities of which are listening and telling stories. As stories are central to the therapeutic relationship and a vital part of qualitative research, then I shall develop below the concept of *narrative* (Aldridge 2000).

Health-care narratives: context and meaning

Spiritual meanings are linked to actions and those actions have consequences that are performed as prayer, meditation, worship and healing. What patients think about the causes of their illnesses influences what they do in terms of health-care treatment and to whom they turn for the resolution of distress. What we have to ask, as health-care practitioners, is does the inclusion of spirituality bring advantages to understanding the people who come to us in distress? As soon as we talk about life being something which we can cherish and preserve, that compassion for others plays an important role in the way in which we choose to live with each other, that service to our communities is a vital activity for maintaining well-being, that hope is an important factor in recovery, then we have the basis for an argument that is spiritual as well as scientific. Essentially I am arguing for a plurality of research understanding in healing. How do we make meaningful connections that form the narratives we make as patients and practitioners, and how do those narratives inform each other?

Anecdotes, the applied language of healing

CAM approaches are often dismissed as relying upon anecdotal material, as if stories are unreliable. My argument is that stories are reliable and rich in information. While we as medical scientists may try and dismiss the anecdote, we rely upon it when we wish to explain particular cases to our colleagues away from the conference podium (Aldridge 1991a, Aldridge 1991b).

Anecdotes may be considered bad science but they are the everyday stuff of clinical practice. People tell us their stories and expect to be heard. Stories have a structure and are told in a style that informs us too. It is not solely the content of a story, it is how it is told that convinces us of its validity. While questionnaires gather information about populations and view the world from the perspective of the researcher, it is the interview that provides the condition for patients to generate their meaningful story. The relationship is the context for the story and patients' stories may change according to the conditions in which they are related. This raises significant validity problems for questionnaire research. Anecdotes are the very stuff of social life and the fabric of communication in the healing encounter. Miller writes that every time the experimental psychologist writes a research report in which anecdotal evidence has been assiduously avoided, the experimental scientist is generating anecdotal evidence for the consumption of his or her colleagues (Miller 1998). The research report itself is an anecdotal report.

Stories play an important role in the healing process, and testimony is an important consideration. Indeed, we have to trust each other in what we say. This is the basis of human communication in the human endeavour of understanding; it is the central plank of qualitative research. When it comes to questions of validity, then we have the concepts of trustworthiness in qualitative research. Testimonies are heard within groups that challenge veracity.

Multiple perspectives

We need a multiple perspective for understanding health-care delivery that is not solely based upon a positivist approach but also upon an interpretative approach. To take such a position is political in that it challenges the major paradigm of scientific research in medicine, a paradigm that is often transparent to those involved. Quite rightly, the qualitative paradigm is also seen as being *critical*; it challenges both the power and privilege of a dominant scientific ideology (Aldridge 1991a, Aldridge 1991b, Aldridge 1991c, Aldridge 1992, Trethewey 1997).

An advantage of qualitative research is that it allows us to see how particular practices are being used. We can discover the meanings attached to activities as they are embedded in day-to-day living. The terms 'healing', 'spirituality', 'intentional' and 'energy' are subject to dictionary definition but also defined by their practice. Qualitative research helps us to understand how such terms are understood in practice (Aldridge 2004a) and that is a political activity, as the feminist movement has reminded us (Aldridge 2004a). We have the right to call our experiences by what terms we wish without a dominant group telling us how that term 'should' be used. While many of us may question the use of the term 'energy' in healing, the word is used by both patients and healers alike, and we might be better directed to discovering its use in practice if we wish to understand it better. When we come to discuss the meaning of healing itself, what role spirituality has in health care, the nature of intentionality, then we are discussing the role of meaning in people's lives. One way to discover those meanings is to ask the participants. The rigour of the asking and the way those meanings are interpreted is the scientific method – *methodology* – of qualitative research.

To understand the health implications of prayer, for example, we can discern the effect of prayer by experiment. However, the impact of prayer from a spiritual perspective is better understood in its subjective interpretation as a qualitative study; both complement each other. If we successfully argue for *complementary* medicine, that is increasingly being called an *integrative* medicine, then surely we can have a congruent paradigm for health-care research that is also complementary and integrative.

A way of seeing how these differing perspectives can be applied to a common problem would be to study those patients who fail to complete a course of treatment, what is sometimes referred to as 'non-compliance'. A positivist paradigm may hypothesise that compliance with the prescribed treatment regime is a matter of patient education. By designing a patient education programme to raise an understanding of the treatment, compliance would be improved according to specific criteria for evaluation. We could design an experiment that would randomise identified non-complying patients to a taught education programme, a leaflet education programme and to no education. Their compliance with medication could then be measured by an assessor blind to the education programme itself.

A qualitative approach would not initially set up an experiment, nor would it try to measure anything. In this instance we would be interested in the experience of patients consulting a practitioner, listening to what the practitioners say, prescribe and advise, and then ask whether patients have complied with that advice. We would be asking where, when, with whom and on what grounds is the decision made not to comply with medical advice. In this case it is the perspective of the non-complier that is as important as the practitioner. Similarly, we may ask patients who also complete a course of treatment and compare them with those who fail to complete. This includes interviews, observations in various settings such as the consulting room and the home, and maybe written material such as diaries. Once we knew the circumstances of non-complying, then we could design suitable initiatives to investigate experimentally. Non-compliance may be located in the patient; it may be a located in the practitioner; or it may be an artefact of their relationship. Unless we discern with whom and when, then our experimental work will be inevitably limited.

From a *critical* research perspective, we would be interested in how a clinic is so organised that some groups fail to have their treatment needs met and where some patterns of treatment response are endemic. This may mean a collaborative inquiry with a self-help patient group and entail some form of advocacy between the clinic and the group (Aldridge 1987d, Reason and Rowan 1981). This latter approach reflects the strong participatory action component of early social-science research.

In order to further illustrate the role of a qualitative perspective for CAM research it is first necessary to provide a brief (and potted) overview of the broad field. Qualitative research is an umbrella term. Some qualitative approaches lean towards an emphasis on analysing texts and interviews (such as content analysis and discourse analysis), while others rely upon descriptions of interaction, that may use a variety of media, and are based upon, ethnography, ethnomethodology, symbolic interactionism and phenomenology. Some qualitative approaches set out to build theories while others aim to discover a particular historical background and locate this within an ideological or political perspective – the assimilation of acupuncture within modern Western medicine, for example, contrasting its acceptance in various European states.

Qualitative research as constructed meanings in context

Qualitative research covers a variety of approaches, and a selection of these is outlined in the following section. What characterises these approaches is an emphasis on understanding the meaning of social activities as they occur in their natural contexts. These are interchangeably called field studies, ethnographies, naturalistic inquiries and case studies. A central plank of these approaches is that we can discern the meaning of social behaviour such as healing and prayer from the experiences that people have in particular contexts, and that these meanings themselves are constructed. Constructed, in the sense that people *make* sense of what they do. The difficulty these approaches face, from a perspective of positivist science, is that because sense is continually being made, and this sense may vary from context to context, there are no universally applicable laws of human behaviour but a series of locally constructed meanings in specific contexts where cultures of healing exist.

Participant observation

Participant observation is a generic term for a qualitative approach where the researcher observes what is happening from an insider position. Rather than administering a set of pre-formed interviews, the participant observer works alongside the staff and patients asking what is going on and listening to what is spontaneously said. Julia Lawton (1998) worked directly alongside patients, their families and staff in the hospice setting to see what was happening. She observed 280 different patients in an intensive study of the dying patient and the dying process in an attempt to answer why some patients are admitted to hospital and others are not. She found that patients are admitted to hospice when bodies begin to disintegrate such that contemporary concepts of the hygienic, sanitised, bounded body become challenged. This builds on the original works of Glaser and Strauss who studied the process of dying (1967). What Lawton does is to challenge the homogenous concept of the hospice as a place for the dying patient and the dying process. She sees the hospice as a place where marginalised cancer patients are referred when they experience difficult symptoms and their bodies deteriorate beyond a socially acceptable boundary. This reflects the challenging nature of qualitative research where what we find out potentially rocks the boat.

Narrative analysis

Researchers from a wide variety of disciplines have found narratives to be useful explaining cross-level psychological phenomena. Narratives with different sources and functions occur at group level and as individual levels of analysis. Research on narratives is particularly useful for understanding the relationship between social process and individual experience, especially in spiritually based communities (Aldridge 1986, Aldridge 1987a, Aldridge 1987b, Aldridge 1987d). Narratives in spiritual settings appear to serve a variety of functions in community life. They define community and facilitate personal change (Aldridge 1987c). As such, local community narratives are vital psychological resources, particularly where dominant cultural narratives fail to adequately represent the lived experience of individuals.

In a family-based treatment approach for suicidal behaviour (Aldridge 1998), what the patient tells as a story, and the narratives of those involved with the patient, generates an important base for treatment initiatives, as well as providing an important source of research material. When analysing family narratives of illness, it was possible to identify specific family features that led to suicidal behaviour: a situation where a family was about to change (by someone leaving or joining), where the identified patient could only do wrong (even when they tried to put things right), and where that person has always been the 'sickly' member of the family. Personal narratives, while being individual, are also located within family narratives, which themselves are located within social contexts. However, these narratives are not accessible to a questionnaire approach; people have to tell them to a listener as a story. It is in the telling that the story gains its strength and meaning; a questionnaire structures information for a different perspective, that of the researcher.

As we have seen earlier, the understanding of patients' stories is vital. Stories, in the hospice, offer the context for elucidating hidden meanings. Little et al. (1998) investigated the illness narratives of patients who had undergone colectomy for colorectal cancer. They asked patients to tell the story of their illness from its first intimations, in their own words with minimal prompting. These interviews were then transcribed and analysed using a grounded-theory approach. From this observational material emerged two phases of subjective experience. An initial phase of disorientation and a sense of loss of control followed by an enduring adaptive phase where the patients constructed and reconstructed their experience through narrative. This last phase they call 'liminality', a dynamic process of adapting to the experience of being ill as expressed in a narrative account of a body that must accommodate the disease and the self.

Potts (1996) examined the role of spirituality in the cancer experiences of sixteen African Americans living in the southern USA. Without any investigator-initiated mention of spirituality, participants referred to many categories of spiritual beliefs and practices that were relevant in their experiences with cancer. When spirituality was specifically explored, there was an even greater elaboration on the initial categories. Key findings included a belief in God as the source of healing, the value of prayer as an instrumental practice, a strategy termed 'turning it over to the Lord', and locating the cancer experience within the context of a greater life narrative. The willingness of care providers to address spiritual and cultural dimensions of cancer enhances therapeutic relationships and the efficacy of psychosocial interventions.

Such narratives are not only important for understanding the process of a disease; they can also make an important contribution to understanding what helps in the process of recovery (Aldridge 1998, Garrett 1997, Spencer et al. 1997). If we are engaged in countering hopelessness as a precursor to failing health, then surely the narratives of patients, and the understandings that we can glean from them, are important factors for consideration in health care and CAM research?

Ethnographic studies

Qualitative researchers are often engaged in fieldwork. They have to physically visit the people in the clinic, their homes, the hospital ward, the street or the village. The forms of documentation necessary for these studies too will vary. Anthropologists have pioneered these methods in learning about other cultures and other cultures of healing. At the heart of these approaches is an emphasis on the researcher being a primary instrument in the research process for the collection of data and for analysing that data. Researchers are involved in the context in which they work; there is an expectation that they are sensitive to non-verbal communication and that they will be interpreting what they experience. These will be referred to here as ethnographic studies.

For example, in a study of mental disorder in Zimbabwe (Patel et al. 1995), 110 subjects were selected by general nurses in three clinics and by four traditional healers from their current clients. The subjects were interviewed using an interview schedule. Mental disorder most commonly presented with somatic symptoms; few patients denied that their mind or soul was the source of illness; and spiritual factors were frequently cited as causes of mental illness. Subjects who were selected by a traditional healer reported a greater duration of illness and were more likely to provide a spiritual explanation for their illness. Most patients, however, showed a mixture of psychiatric symptoms that did not fall clearly into a single diagnostic group, and patients with a spiritual model of illness were less likely to conform to criteria of 'caseness' and represented a unique category of psychological distress in Zimbabwe.

The significance of healing rituals is important for understanding how health care may best be implemented. An ethnographic study of a church-based healing clinic in Jamaica (Griffith 1983) shows how mixing spiritual, psychological and conventional medical needs, with their heterodox beliefs and values, creates tension. While a new ritual format needed to be introduced, it is difficult to transform traditional formats of healing. Such an ethnographic qualitative perspective could be used to discern how CAM approaches are used within modern healing cultures within health-care clinics.

Phenomenology

While experience and interpretation are at the heart of all qualitative methods, there are also particular phenomenological approaches that look to the essence of a structure or an experience. The assumption that an essence to an experience exists is similar to the assumption by an ethnographer that culture exists. Prior beliefs are first identified and then temporarily set aside so that the phenomenon being studied may be seen in a new light. In a study of the phenomenon of prayer we would want to know what constitutes the consciousness of praying, what the sensory experiences of prayer are, what our thoughts are and what emotions are involved. Setting and context would also be central to this phenomenological understanding. In this way, we see that investigating the lives of mystics would provide documentary evidence of a phenomenological understanding of prayer and meditation.

Phenomenological studies are well suited to understanding the world of the sufferer. An interpretative phenomenological study, which began as a study of the meaning of being restrained, offers a glimpse into mental illness (Johnson 1998). Ten psychiatric patients were interviewed and the audio-taped interviews transcribed. The resulting texts were analysed using a process methodology developed from Heideggerian hermeneutical phenomenology. Two major themes emerged: 'struggling' and 'why me?', revealing what it was like for the participants to live with a serious mental illness. As part of their struggling, patients asked the existential question 'Why me?', a question repeatedly heard when working with the dying. This study underscores how important it is for the therapist caring for a patient to enter into, and try to understand, the world of that patient – a position that emphasises the practical application of qualitative research for CAM practice.

Grounded theory

Qualitative research attempts to glean understandings from experience. This is not theory testing but theory generation and is used where existing theories fail to explain the phenomenon satisfactorily. Given that placebo, for example, is a concept in common use by practitioners, qualitative researchers would ask, and observe, those practitioners when they believed placebo to be occurring and what they understood a placebo practice to be. Similarly, qualitative researchers would also ask patients about their understandings of what is happening. This breaks the cycle of abstract definitions being brokered amongst scientists and locates explanations in everyday practices. In this way, theories are generated that match the data gathered from experience and this has led to the approach known as 'grounded theory' (Strauss and Corbin 1990). Grounded theory elucidates substantive theories applicable to understanding localised practices that have a high internal and content validity, rather than grand theories of medicine.

Research in healing

Modern science implies that there is a common map of the territory of healing, with particular coordinates and given symbols for finding our way around, and that the map of scientific medicine is our sole guide. We need to recognise that scientific medicine emphasises one particular way of knowing amongst others. Scientific thinking maintains the myth that to know anything we must be scientists; however, people who live in vast desert areas find their way across trackless terrain without any understandings of scientific geography. They also know the pattern of the weather without recourse to what we know as the science of meteorology.

In a similar way, people know about their own bodies and have understandings about their own lives without the benefit of anatomy or psychology. They may not confer the same meanings on their experiences of health and illness as we researchers do, yet it is towards an understanding of personal and idiosyncratic beliefs to which we might most wisely be guiding our research endeavours. By understanding the stories people tell us of their healing and the insights this brings, then we may begin to truly understand the efficacy of a range of CAM. That health and the divine are brought together in such spiritualities as prayer is a challenge for renewal of our understanding in health care and not grounds for dismissal as invalid.

When we speak of scientific or experimental validity, we speak of a validity that has to be conferred by a person or group of persons on the work or actions of another group. This is a 'political' process. With the obsession for 'objective truths' in the scientific community other 'truths' are ignored. As clinicians we have many ways of knowing: by intuition, through experience and by observation. If we disregard these 'knowings' then we promote the idea that there is an objective definitive external truth that exists as 'tablets of stone' and to which only we, the initiated, have access.

The people with whom clinicians work in the therapist–patient relationship are not experimental units. Nor are the measurements made on these people separate and independent sets of data. While at times it may be necessary to treat the data as independent of the person, we must make such processes explicit when we come to measure particular personal variables in order to avoid complications. The clinical measurements of blood status, weight and temperature are important. However, they belong to a different realm of understanding than do issues of anxiety about the future, the experience of pain, the anticipation of personal and social losses and the existential feeling of abandonment. These defy comparative measurement. Yet if we are to investigate therapeutic approaches to chronic disease, we need to investigate these subjective and qualitative realms. While we may be able to make little change in blood status, we can take heed of emotional status and propose initiatives for treatment. The goal of therapy (CAM or otherwise) is not always to cure, it can also be to comfort and relieve. The involvement of the physician with the biologic dimension of disease has resulted in an amnesia for the necessary understanding of suffering in the patient (Cassell 1991).

In the same way, we can achieve changes in existential states through prayer and meditation, the evidence for which can only be metaphorically expressed and humanly witnessed. Are we to impoverish our culture by denying that this happens and discounting what people tell us? What then are we to trust in our lives, the dialogue with our friends or the displays of our machines? This is not an argument against technology. It is an argument for narrative and relationship in understanding what it is to be human – that is, the basis for *qualitative* research in CAM.

In terms of outcomes measurement, we face further difficulties. The people we see in our clinics do not live in isolation. Life is rather a messy laboratory and continually influences the subjects of our therapeutic and research endeavours. The way people respond in situations is sometimes determined by the way in which they have understood the meaning of that situation. The meaning of hair loss, weight loss, loss of potency, loss of libido, impending death and the nature of suffering will be differently perceived in varying cultures. To this balding, ageing researcher, hair loss is a fact of life. My Greek neighbour says that if it happens to him it will be a disaster. When we deliver a powerful therapeutic agent we are not treating an isolated example of a clinical entity but intervening in an ecology of responses and beliefs which are somatic, psychological, social and spiritual.

In a similar way, what Western medicine understands as surgery, intubation and medication others may perceive as mutilation, invasion and poison. Cultural differences regarding the integrity of the body will influence ethical issues such as abortion and body transplants. Treatment initiatives may be standardised in terms of the culture of the administrating researchers, but the perceptions of the subjects of the research, and their families, may be incongruous and various. Actually, we know from studies of treatment options in breast cancer that physicians beliefs also vary, and these beliefs influence the information the physicians give to their patients (Ganz 1992). If we return to the concepts of placebo and non-compliance, then it is surely a qualitative research paradigm that will encourage a practical understanding of the patient–practitioner relationship.

Difficulties in researching prayer and spiritual healing

We know that there are major difficulties with intentional healing research. Achieving transcendence, an understanding of purpose and meaning is an activity. It occurs in a relationship and that is informed by culture. Research initiatives that concentrate on the healer fail to understand the activity of the patient, lose sight of the relationship and ignore the cultural factors involved. I am using 'culture' here to refer to the system of symbolic meanings that are available, not demographic data. Losing this nesting of contexts fragments the healing endeavour, emphasising a passive patient that receives healing rather that an active patient participating in a common enterprise. A qualitative approach to CAM emphasises the involvement of the patient and approaches healing as a relational activity.

Much research is carried out using a conventional medical-science paradigm to understand spiritual healing and prayer, but the intention of that research is not always made clear (Aldridge 2000). If the intention is to demonstrate the efficacy of spiritual healing approaches and prayer, then the methodology is clearly misguided. I suspect that much of this research is not being carried out for patients but as a strategy in the politics of establishing alternative healing initiatives within conventional medical approaches. Therefore we have healing groups promoting their own interest and adopting the methodological approach of randomised clinical trials considered to be suitable for acceptance rather than looking at what is necessary for discovering what is happening. This is not to say that the results of clinical randomised trials are not influential, rather that they are limited in their applicability as far as prayer and healing are to be understood if:

- the patient is expected to be active;
- there has to be a relationship with the healer;
- there are no definite end-points in time;
- healing can appear as differing phenomena;
- and the prayer has to be non-specific and non-directional.

(See Pirotta, Chapter 4, for more details of the application of RCT to CAM and Verhoef and Vanderheyden, Chapter 5, for a discussion of the mixing of qualitative methods and RCTs.)

Healing, like prayer, is not a homogenous practice and is not susceptible to standardisation. Attempts at standardisation would no longer make it prayer but superstitious incantation or magical hand passes. Relationship is central and while faith may not be necessary, the engagement of the patient is fundamental. The ability to heal is seen in some traditions as a divine gift; it may not be available to all and even to those that have the gift not available all of the time (Aldridge 2000). Ascertaining who has it, and when, is not easy. Healing is also considered, in some traditions, to be a secondary ability of spiritual development that can be systematically applied, but it is an advanced ability (Aldridge 2000). This again proves to be a difficulty, as presumably there are more practitioners with lower abilities than advanced practitioners that are more reliable in their efficacy. And who in the world of healing practitioners is going to say that they are less advanced? Those who are advanced in such understandings will probably see no need to subject such knowledge to material worldly proof.

Indeed, we must return to the purpose of proof. We see already that spiritual healing is practised and that medical practitioners refer to such healers. If the grounds of research are for payment or to institute professional practice then maybe the results will be elusive as opposed to when the purpose is for the pursuit and improvement of human knowledge. One system of knowledge cannot be predicated on proofs from another system of knowledge.

Conclusion

> It would be wrong to permit medicine to use the authority it has gained from scientific and technical proficiency . . . as a cloak to gain authority over questions that most in society consider moral and religious.
>
> (Smolin 1995)

When people come to their practitioners (CAM and others), they are asking about what will become of them. What will their future be like? Will there be a change? Some practitioners make a prognosis based on the interview that they have had with the patient. Sometimes this will be the dreaded answer to the question 'How long do I have to live?' But with each interview there is the question of when healing will take place. What can be expected in the near future, and is there any hope of a cure? The story of what happens is, in part, a clinical history. It is also no less than the narration of destiny, the unfolding of a person's life purpose (Larner 1998). When we talk with the dying, it is this sense of purpose, 'Was it all worthwhile?', that is a critical moment in coping with the situation. The telling and listening, the *relating* of these stories, is the very stuff of qualitative research.

Stories are the recounting of what happens in time. They are not simply located in the past but are also about real events that happen now and what expectations there are for the future. Tellers are active agents. They are not passively experiencing their past but performing an identity with another person. That other person as doctor, priest or healer has the moral obligation through the therapeutic contract to listen and engage in the healing relationship. Stories are told. They are not simply private accounts that we relate to ourselves, they have a public function and will vary according to whom is listening and the way in which the listeners are reacting. Qualitative research has incorporated such narratives into its approach to understanding health care (Strauss and Corbin 1990, Aldridge 1998, Hall 1998, van Manen 1998).

Narratives bring a coherence and order to life stories – stories make sense. Yet the scientific null hypothesis assumes, at the very core of its reasoning, that there is no such coherence (Larner 1998). Technology strives to domesticate time as *chronos*, to make time even and predictable. We can approach time as *kairos*, uneven, biological and decisive, in that the moment must be seized (Aldridge 1996). This makes a mockery of fixed outcomes in that the time and logic of healing may have modes elusive to commercialised requirements of health-care delivery. Peace of mind may occur but no cure. Forgiveness may take place but no change in survival time. Are we really to throw away such outcomes of peace of mind and forgiveness because they find no immediate material expression? Perhaps it is the very denial of those qualities that provokes the restlessness of people today as they seek an elusive state of health despite the material riches of Western cultures.

No material change may occur in spiritual healing, but the individuals transcend their immediate situation. Furthermore, there are no personal stories in medical science but group probabilities. This is seriously at odds with the demands of the patients' encounter with their doctor or therapist, which is personal. People are subjective. They are indeed subjects, and subjects that need to relate a story to another person that understands them. To be treated as objects in a world of social events deprives them of meaning. It is this very lack of meaning that exacerbates suffering. When people come to practitioners for treatment they have an expectation that tomorrow will bring something different from today, not the expectation of a probability that tomorrow will be the same as today.

Becoming sick, being treated, achieving recovery and becoming well are plots in the narrative of life. As such they are a reminder of our mortality. They are a historical relationship; meanings are linked together in time. Stories have a shape, they have purpose, and they are bounded in time. Thus, we talk about a case history. It is for this reason that group studies fail to offer an essential understanding of what it is to fall ill and become well. Generalisation loses individual intent and time is removed. The individual biographical historicity is lost in favour of the group. Purpose and intent are important in life, they are at the basis of hope. If that purpose is abandoned through hopelessness, then suicide and death are the outcome. In our healing endeavours we need to consider the circumstances in which healing occurs and how those circumstances are enabled. This is not the technological approach of cure but the ecological approach of providing the ground in which healing is achieved, whether it be an organic, psychological, social or spiritual context. Those healing contexts will also be part of a biography; they have an historicity, and this must be included too in our research.

At the heart of much scientific thinking in the medical world is a desire for prediction and to base treatment strategies and outcomes on a group statistic of probability (Aldridge 2004a). This is quite rightly explained as the desire to provide the optimum treatment and to eliminate false treatment that harms. Such a statement too is based upon belief, a touching faith in statistical reasoning. Behind this thinking is an assumption that tomorrow will be the same as today and that the future is predicated on the past. What many of our patients hope, and the purpose of our endeavours in both CAM practice and research, is that tomorrow will be new. Qualitative research methods are one way of discovering the new in the way in which we tell our stories together.

References

Aldridge, D. (1986) 'Licence to heal', *Crucible*, April–June: 58–66.
—— (1987a) 'A community approach to cancer in families', *Journal of Maternal and Child Health*, 12: 182–5.
—— (1987b) 'Families, cancer and dying', *Family Practice*, 4 (3): 212–18.
—— (1987c) *One Body: A Guide to Healing in the Church*, London: SPCK.
—— (1987d) 'A team approach to terminal care: personal implications for patients and practitioners', *Journal of the Royal College of General Practitioners*, 37 (301): 364.
—— (1991a) 'Aesthetics and the individual in the practice of medical research: a discussion paper', *Journal of the Royal Society of Medicine*, 84 (3): 147–50.
—— (1991b) 'Healing and medicine', *Journal of the Royal Society of Medicine*, 84 (9): 516–18.
—— (1991c) 'Spirituality, healing and medicine', *Journal of British General Practice*, 41 (351): 425–7.
—— (1992) 'The needs of individual patients in clinical research', *Advances*, 8 (4): 58–65.
—— (1996) *Music Therapy Research and Practice in Medicine: From Out of the Silence*, London: Jessica Kingsley.
—— (1998) *Suicide: The Tragedy of Hopelessness*, London: Jessica Kingsley.
—— (2000) *Spirituality, Healing and Medicine*, London: Jessica Kingsley.
—— (2004a) *The Individual, Health and Integrated Medicine: In Search of an Health Care Aesthetic*, London: Jessica Kingsley.
—— (2004b) 'The reflective practitioner in a community of inquiry: case study designs', *Journal of Holistic Healthcare*, 1 (2): 19–23.
Cassell, E. (1991) *The Nature of Suffering and the Goals of Medicine*, New York: Oxford University Press.
Cornelius, J. B. (1999) 'The meaning of AIDS: African American nursing students' perceptions of providing care to AIDS patients', *Journal of National Black Nurses Association*, 10 (2): 54–64.
Denzin, N. K. and Lincoln, Y. S. (1994) *Handbook of Qualitative Research*, London: Sage.
Dorozario, L. (1997) 'Spirituality in the lives of people with disability and chronic illness: a creative paradigm of wholeness and reconstitution', *Disability and Rehabilitation*, 19 (1): 427–34.
Dossey, L. (1993) *Healing Words: The Power of Prayer and the Practice of Medicine*, New York: Harper Collins.
Ganz, P. (1992) 'Treatment options for breast cancer-beyond survival', *The New England Journal of Medicine*, 326 (17): 1147–9.
Garrett, C. J. (1997) 'Recovery from anorexia nervosa: a sociological perspective', *International Journal of Eating Disorders*, 21 (3): 261–72.
Glaser, B. and Strauss, A. (1967) *The Discovery of Grounded Theory*, Chicago, Ill.: Aldine.
Griffith, E. (1983) 'The significance of ritual in a church-based healing model', *American Journal of Psychiatry*, 140 (5): 568–72.
Hall, B. (1998) 'Patterns of spirituality in persons with advanced HIV disease', *Research in Nursing and Health*, 21 (2): 143–53.

Johnson, M. E. (1998) 'Being mentally ill: a phenomenological inquiry' *Archives of Psychiatric Nursing*, 12: 195–201.

Kleinman, A. (1973) 'Medicine's symbolic reality: on a central problem in the philosophy of medicine', *Inquiry*, 16: 206–13.

Larner, G. (1998) 'Through a glass darkly', *Theory and Psychology*, 8 (4): 549–72.

Lawton, J. (1998) 'Contemporary hospice care: the sequestration of the unbounded body and "dirty dying" ', *Sociology of Health and Illness*, 20 (2): 121–43.

Lewinsohn, R. (1998) 'Medical theories, science, and the practice of medicine', *Social Science and Medicine*, 46 (10): 1261–70.

Little, M., Jordens, C., Paul, K., Montgomery, K. and Philipson, B. (1998) 'Liminality: a major category of the experience of cancer illness', *Social Science and Medicine*, 47 (10): 1485–94.

Mechanic, D. (1968) *Medical Sociology*, New York: The Free Press.

Miller, R. (1998) 'Epistemology and psychotherapy data: the unspeakable, unbearable, horrible truth', *Clinical Psychology: Science and Practice*, 5 (2): 242–50.

Patel, V., Gwanzura, F., Simunyu, E., Lloyd, K. and Mann, A. (1995) 'The phenomenology and explanatory models of common mental disorder: a study in primary care in Harare, Zimbabwe', *Psychological Medicine*, 25 (6): 1191–9.

Potts, R. (1996) 'Spirituality and the experience of cancer in an African-American community: implications for psychosocial oncology', *Journal of Psychosocial Oncology*, 14 (1): 1–19.

Reason, P. and Rowan, J. (1981) *Human Inquiry*, Chichester: John Wiley.

Smolin, D. (1995) 'Praying for baby Rena: religious liberty, medical futility, and miracles', *Seton Hall Law Review*, 25: 960–96.

Spencer, J., Davidson, H. and White, V. (1997) 'Helping clients develop hopes for the future', *American Journal of Occupational Therapy*, 51 (3): 191–8.

Strauss, A. and Corbin, J. (1990) *Basics of Qualitative Research: Grounded Theory Procedures and Techniques*, Newbury Park, Calif.: Sage.

Trethewey, A. (1997) 'Resistance, identity, and empowerment: a postmodern feminist analysis of clients in a human service organization', *Communication Monographs*, 64 (4): 281–301.

Van Manen, M. (1998) 'Modalities of body experience in illness and health', *Qualitative Health Research*, 8 (1): 7–24.

Williams, C., Wilson, C. and Olsen, C. (2005) 'Dying, death, and medical education: student voices', *Journal of Palliative Medicine*, 8 (2): 372–81.

Chapter 2

Systematic reviews and CAM

Eric Manheimer and Jeanette Ezzo

Introduction

Most systematic reviews of CAM restrict inclusion to RCTs, widely regarded as the most unbiased study design for evaluating health-care interventions. Systematic reviewers evaluate and synthesise RCTs using objective, transparent and reproducible methods in order to assess the overall effects of a given therapy and systematic reviews sometimes include a meta-analysis, the quantitative combining (pooling) of results from similar but separate RCTs to obtain an overall effect estimate.

Over the past twenty-five years, there has been an explosion in the number of meta-analyses in CAM (Figure 2.1). Meta-analysis now has the greatest citation impact of all study designs (exceeding even RCTs) and is continuing to increase (Patsopoulos et al. 2005). This citation impact of meta-analysis/systematic review is also commensurate with its position at the top of the hierarchy of research evidence (Atkins et al. 2004) and the recent interest in CAM from the Cochrane Collaboration (Manheimer and Berman 2005) (as of July 2005, there were 2,435 completed Cochrane reviews and more than 150 CAM-related Cochrane reviews). This chapter provides an overview of systematic review methods in relation to CAM, summarises current research on CAM systematic reviews and illustrates through case examples various approaches used to address methodological challenges in CAM reviews.

Systematic reviews: their importance to research

Systematic reviews are rapidly becoming the cornerstone of evidence-based medicine with clinicians ranking reviews as the primary source of new information (Lehmann and Goodman 1995). Policy-makers increasingly rely on systematic reviews as a way of summarising evidence (Dickersin and Manheimer 1998) and consumers use reviews to guide health decisions (Bero and Jadad 1997).

Information from systematic reviews also aid researchers in their attempts

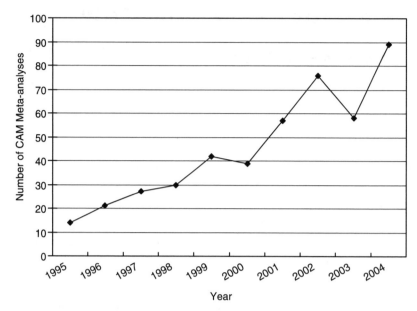

Figure 2.1 Number of CAM meta-analyses indexed on PubMed, 1995–2004.*

*This search was performed on October 14, 2005 using the following search strategy to obtain counts for each year: CAM [Subset] AND meta-analysis [Publication Type] AND *year* [Date of Publication]. There is no Medline Publication Type term for *systematic review* and as a consequence we used the Publication Type term *meta-analysis* as an indicator for tracking growth in interest in systematic reviews over the past ten years. While the term *meta-analysis* is likely to have a high precision in identifying systematic reviews (because a meta-analysis is generally also a systematic review), this term is likely to have only a low to moderate sensitivity because many systematic reviews do not include a meta-analysis.

to plan clinical trials. The systematic review serves to ensure that the proposed trial is relevant, necessary and guided by earlier trials. Amidst the vast, almost limitless, number of research questions that remain to be addressed in CAM, and the limited financial support available to study non-proprietary CAM therapies, it is important that researchers plan their trials in the context of what is already known on a topic. Having spent months studying the existing CAM trials, systematic reviewers are well versed in the strengths and weaknesses of current trials and often ideally suited to suggest methodological improvements for future trials. For example, Berman et al. (2004) designed a large, phase III 'acupuncture for knee osteoarthritis' trial using guidelines from an earlier review (Ezzo et al. 2001) and McNeely et al. (2004) cite the methodological limitations of an earlier systematic review as a stimulus for their recent research design.

Systematic reviews have a two-way, iterative relationship with clinical trials, and this is well illustrated with the example of acupuncture for low back pain.

The earliest Cochrane review of trials on this topic was inconclusive due to methodological weaknesses (van Tulder et al. 1999). Larger, more rigorous trials were conducted, addressing the issues raised in the Cochrane review, and the two most recent systematic reviews of acupuncture for low back pain (Furlan et al. 2005, Manheimer et al. 2005) conducted by two independent research teams both show positive findings favouring acupuncture compared to control for chronic low back pain.

Systematic reviews can also influence primary research by suggesting priorities for investigation. Some reviews now include suggestions for high-priority research based on known mechanisms of action and safety. For example, a review of CAM for dementia cited huperzine A, levacecarnine, and EGB 761 as warranting further examination based on the methodological quality of the studies, mechanisms of action and overall safety (Diamond et al. 2003).

Systematic reviews require rigorous methods

Systematic reviews can be prone to the biases that also plague other research study designs. In the context of systematic reviews, the term 'bias' is used to designate some systematic study-related error resulting in the failure to reflect the real world association between treatment and outcome. The susceptibility to bias within systematic reviews is illustrated in a number of ways. First, systematic review findings have occasionally been overturned by the findings of large, well-designed RCTs (LeLorier et al. 1997). Second, as Linde and Willich (2003) illustrate with regard to acupuncture, herbal medicine and homoeopathy, systematic reviews that address the same research question sometimes employ different methods of review leading to differences in results and conclusions. Systematic reviews are designed to ensure rigorous quality standards and maintain objectivity during each phase of review preparation, including: (1) identifying relevant RCTs; (2) assessing the quality of the RCTs; and (3) combining the data from the RCTs. Issues regarding these three items are discussed in the following three sections.

Identifying relevant trials

Conducting a thorough, well-documented search for trials is one of the key elements that distinguishes a systematic review from a traditional narrative review. While comprehensive searches of multiple-database and non-database sources of all languages are ideal under optimal circumstances, such far-reaching searches are not always practical given time and budget constraints. As a result, thoroughness needs to be balanced with efficiency. The best way to achieve this balance is to be aware of, and aim to minimise, the various biases that can result from restricting searches in different ways.

Can searches be restricted to major databases?

Research examining searches restricted to only the US National Library of Medicine's Medline database (or Medline and other major databases) shows these methods yield non-comprehensive results. Medline sensitivity averaged 51 per cent (range 17–82 per cent), for a sample of studies including both CAM and conventional medicine topics, even when databases were searched by a trained searcher (Dickersin et al. 1994).

When searches are restricted to only trials in journals available on Medline, a substantial proportion (23 per cent) remain unidentified due to the inconsistent terminology employed to index randomised trials (Dickersin et al. 1994). Such indexing difficulties have been documented for acupuncture trials (Pilkington and Richardson 2004) and CAM trials more generally (Murphy et al. 2003).

More current research on locating trials is pertinent given that indexing, coverage of databases and trial reporting have all improved in recent years (Begg et al. 1996). A particular problem regarding CAM RCTs, which are often published in low-impact journals that are not a high indexing priority, is indexing lag time. For example, while extensive searches beyond the major databases have been shown to be necessary to identify nine of the twenty-one RCTs included in a systematic review of acupuncture (Savoie et al. 2003), post-hoc analysis shows that most of these RCTs have been indexed in the major databases one year later.

Other CAM researchers, conducting a systematic review of nutritional dietary supplements for patients after hip fracture, have evaluated the yield of RCTs by supplementing major database searches with other searches (for example, contacting experts, hand searching journals) (Avenell et al. 2001). In this case, a search of only Medline and Embase articles would have missed approximately half of the eligible RCTs for this review. This is not surprising because Medline and Embase often exclude journals (often published in certain countries or languages [Pilkington et al. 2005]) which are likely to report CAM trials. Indeed, the proportion of non-Medline-indexed trials in CAM-related meta-analyses (40.9 per cent) is approximately twice the proportion in conventional medicine meta-analyses (22.4 per cent) (Egger et al. 2003).

Can reviews exclude non-English-language publications?

Research has also examined the impact of including as opposed to excluding non-English-language trials. Such an impact is important because the identification and translation of non-English-language trials will substantially add to the costs of a review and will require the involvement of an international review team.

Several studies have shown, to a greater or lesser degree, that excluding trials published in non-English languages does not appear to substantially change effect estimates in meta-analyses of conventional medicine (Moher et al. 2000, Juni et al. 2002, Egger et al. 2003, Moher et al. 2003). Meanwhile, Moher et al. (2005) have shown that excluding non-English-language trials in CAM meta-analyses does change the effect estimates. The picture remains inconclusive and, ultimately, more research needs to be done to determine whether there are differential publication trends for CAM according to language, country and CAM modality.

Given the lack of a generalisable conclusion about non-English languages and CAM, there is fairly widespread agreement that for CAM, where a substantial proportion of the studies are not included in Medline and other easy to access sources (Pilkington et al. 2005), a non-comprehensive search may miss many eligible trials (Egger et al. 2003). Although the studies that prove difficult to retrieve may be of lower quality (Egger et al. 2003), it has been suggested that the correct approach is to not exclude them, but rather to evaluate their effects on the results of the review using sensitivity analyses (Egger et al. 2003, Moher et al. 2003).

Assessing the methodological quality of RCTs

RCTs are the gold standard for evaluating the effects of health-care therapies. However, the quality of RCTs is not uniform. Lower-quality RCTs result in larger, and presumably inflated, effect estimates compared with RCTs of higher quality (Juni et al. 2001, Egger et al. 2003). As a result, evaluating RCT quality has become a standard component of systematic-reviews methodology (Moja et al. 2005) and this is as important for CAM as for any other area of health-care research. We do not provide a detailed discussion of this area here (for a detailed discussion of RCTs, their applicability and quality with regard to CAM see Pirotta, Chapter 4). However, one issue we would like to contemplate is the reporting of quality in RCT publications.

Quality is generally evaluated based on the information from the RCT publication, thus assuming that what is written in the publication reflects actual study procedure and that 'if it is not reported, it probably was not done.' In conventional medicine, existing studies covering different topic areas and publication periods have had contradictory findings on the utility of contacting investigators to obtain additional, unreported information about trial quality. A summary of the studies is published elsewhere (Manheimer et al. in press).

We recently evaluated this question in CAM by contacting principal investigators of acupuncture RCTs to request information about randomisation and blinding procedures not described in RCT publications (Manheimer et al. in press). The investigation identified that over one-third of the trials had used appropriate random allocation concealment methods, but the investigators had failed to describe the details in their publications. While this survey suggests that contacting CAM trialists may result in obtaining previously unpublished information about methodological quality, the potential gains of obtaining the missing information may be outweighed by the reporting bias such efforts may introduce. Data obtained directly from investigators has not been peer reviewed and may not be as reliable as data extracted from published articles. Inadequate trial reporting is becoming less of a problem as a result of the CONSORT statement (Begg et al. 1996) providing a set of guidelines specifying reporting requirements for RCTs and an adaptation of CONSORT specifically for acupuncture trials, called STRICTA (MacPherson et al. 2002), has been widely disseminated in CAM journals.

Combining the data from RCTs in a meta-analysis: a case study

In deciding whether and how to statistically pool the results of similar but separate RCTs, systematic reviewers must consider the homogeneity of the populations studied, the therapies administered and the control comparisons used, as well as the homogeneity of the design and results of the RCTs. This is well illustrated with the use of a recently conducted systematic review and meta-analysis of acupuncture for low back pain (Manheimer et al. 2005).

Heterogeneity of the trials was an important concern for this systematic review because the effects of acupuncture may vary depending on the style of acupuncture evaluated (Chinese or Western), the type of control comparison (sham, no treatment or another active treatment) and the type of pain in the patients studied (acute or chronic). To address potential heterogeneity, we decided, a priori, that eligible RCTs would be pooled in a meta-analysis only if they tested the same style of acupuncture against the same type of control for patients with the same type of low back pain. It transpired that a majority (twenty-two out of thirty-three) of the RCTs eligible for the systematic review evaluated *Chinese*-style acupuncture for patients with *chronic* low back pain. The results of these RCTs, which were generally of fairly high quality, were meta-analysed together and stratified by control group in the primary analysis.

Figure 2.2 shows the results of this primary analysis, as a forest plot, the standard diagram for presenting meta-analysis results. The structure of the forest plot and the significance of the placement of the horizontal lines will be explained using the example of the sham-acupuncture controlled RCTs, grouped together at the top of the diagram. The horizontal lines associated with three out of four of these sham-acupuncture controlled RCTs did not cross the central vertical line of no effect, which indicates that these three trials all found acupuncture to be statistically significantly better than the sham-acupuncture control. The pooled result of all four of the sham-acupuncture controlled RCTs is indicated by the open circle (signifying

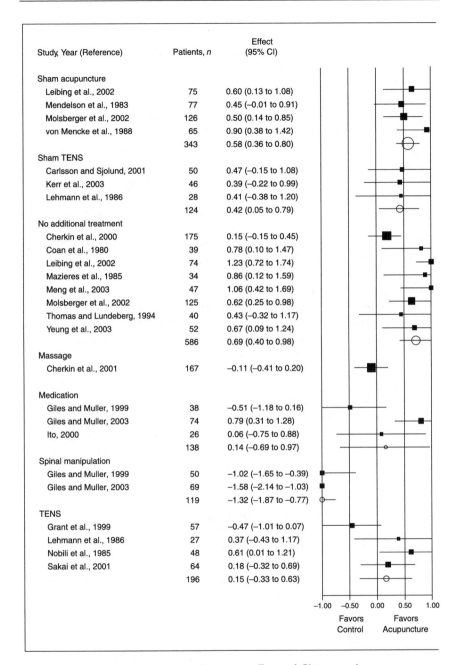

Study, Year (Reference)	Patients, n	Effect (95% CI)	
Sham acupuncture			
Leibing et al., 2002	75	0.60 (0.13 to 1.08)	
Mendelson et al., 1983	77	0.45 (−0.01 to 0.91)	
Molsberger et al., 2002	126	0.50 (0.14 to 0.85)	
von Mencke et al., 1988	65	0.90 (0.38 to 1.42)	
	343	0.58 (0.36 to 0.80)	
Sham TENS			
Carlsson and Sjolund, 2001	50	0.47 (−0.15 to 1.08)	
Kerr et al., 2003	46	0.39 (−0.22 to 0.99)	
Lehmann et al., 1986	28	0.41 (−0.38 to 1.20)	
	124	0.42 (0.05 to 0.79)	
No additional treatment			
Cherkin et al., 2000	175	0.15 (−0.15 to 0.45)	
Coan et al., 1980	39	0.78 (0.10 to 1.47)	
Leibing et al., 2002	74	1.23 (0.72 to 1.74)	
Mazieres et al., 1985	34	0.86 (0.12 to 1.59)	
Meng et al., 2003	47	1.06 (0.42 to 1.69)	
Molsberger et al., 2002	125	0.62 (0.25 to 0.98)	
Thomas and Lundeberg, 1994	40	0.43 (−0.32 to 1.17)	
Yeung et al., 2003	52	0.67 (0.09 to 1.24)	
	586	0.69 (0.40 to 0.98)	
Massage			
Cherkin et al., 2001	167	−0.11 (−0.41 to 0.20)	
Medication			
Giles and Muller, 1999	38	−0.51 (−1.18 to 0.16)	
Giles and Muller, 2003	74	0.79 (0.31 to 1.28)	
Ito, 2000	26	0.06 (−0.75 to 0.88)	
	138	0.14 (−0.69 to 0.97)	
Spinal manipulation			
Giles and Muller, 1999	50	−1.02 (−1.65 to −0.39)	
Giles and Muller, 2003	69	−1.58 (−2.14 to −1.03)	
	119	−1.32 (−1.87 to −0.77)	
TENS			
Grant et al., 1999	57	−0.47 (−1.01 to 0.07)	
Lehmann et al., 1986	27	0.37 (−0.43 to 1.17)	
Nobili et al., 1985	48	0.61 (0.01 to 1.21)	
Sakai et al., 2001	64	0.18 (−0.32 to 0.69)	
	196	0.15 (−0.33 to 0.63)	

−1.00   −0.50   0.00   0.50   1.00

Favors Control   Favors Acupuncture

Figure 2.2 Meta-analysis forest plot: short-term effects of Chinese-style acupuncture on chronic pain.

the effect estimate) intersected by a horizontal line (signifying the confidence interval of this effect estimate).

The diagram indicates that both the sham controlled RCTs and the no-treatment controlled RCTs suggest acupuncture to be an effective treatment for relieving pain in the short term. However, the sham controlled RCTs generally show less benefit of acupuncture compared with the no-treatment controlled RCTs. The less positive outcome in the sham controlled RCTs is not surprising considering the potential for sham controlled RCTs to under-estimate the specific effects of acupuncture (especially if the sham needles are inserted, thereby potentially stimulating a physiologic response) (Paterson and Dieppe 2005) and for no-treatment controlled trials (which are not blinded) to overestimate acupuncture's specific effects.

While the similarities of the RCTs' clinical characteristics, as described above, seemed to justify their pooling across control groups, before actually pooling the data, we also considered the separate but related issue of whether similarity in the statistical results of the RCTs could justify their statistical pooling. If the sham-acupuncture controlled RCTs had wildly different results, for example, then one might question the appropriateness of stat-istical pooling, even if the clinical characteristics of these trials seemed simi-lar. Such pooling would especially be a concern if a difference in results were associated with a difference in design or methodological quality between the trials, for example. In this meta-analysis, we used statistical tests (Deeks et al. 2005) to examine whether the results of the effects of acupuncture versus sham acupuncture were heterogeneous at different levels of any quality (for example, concealed allocation or not), patient (severe pain or not), or treatment-related (for example, number of sessions) criteria. We found that the results of these sham-acupuncture controlled trials were clearly homo-geneous (see Figure 2.2) and no results on heterogeneity tests were positive for any criteria tested. The homogeneity of results (as indicated by the fact that the horizontal lines associated with the sham controlled trials all overlap) strengthened our confidence in both the appropriateness of using meta-analysis in this review and in the results of the review.

As mentioned above, twenty-two of the thirty-three studies in this system-atic review evaluated the same style of acupuncture among patients with the same type of pain and were therefore judged sufficiently homogeneous to pool in our meta-analyses (see Figure 2.2). For the remaining eleven RCTs, which were fundamentally heterogeneous on style of acupuncture, type of pain and control comparison used, we employed a narrative description along with a tabular presentation of study characteristics and results instead of a meta-analysis. We did not meta-analyse any subset of these eleven trials due to the small number of RCTs within each subset, the small sample sizes and often poor reporting and low quality.

CAM systematic reviewers often cannot conduct a meta-analysis because of a dearth of available RCTs or deficiencies in the conduct and reporting of existing RCTs. A best-evidence synthesis is a qualitative alternative to a strictly narrative approach (van Tulder et al. 2003). This method evaluates the consistency, quality and strength of the reviewed RCTs and, based on this evaluation, assigns a therapy a level of evidence: strong, moderate, limited, conflicting or none.

Additional research issues in CAM reviews

CAM reviewers commonly encounter additional methodological challenges. These are often judgement calls – situations where there is not one right answer but where reviewers have to choose one method over another, knowing the imperfections of each. Some common methodological issues include how to address treatment adequacy, practitioner adequacy, cointerventions and safety.

Assessment of the treatment adequacy

The discussion about trial validity in the first part of this chapter pertains to design issues such as concealment and blinding that are common across trials regardless of whether the trial is a drug or a CAM trial. Failure to address these issues can bias the review conclusions predominantly on the side of a type I error (a false-positive finding). However, many CAM interventions lack the dose-finding Phase I and II research of drug trials, and inadequate 'doses' can bias results towards a type II error (a false-negative finding).

Although treatment adequacy should be addressed in clinical trials, systematic reviews need a method for assessing it. Acupuncture reviews provide examples of a variety of ways treatment adequacy has been addressed. One treatment-adequacy assessment first proposed by Linde et al. (1996) involves presenting inclusion criteria and methods sections of acupuncture papers to acupuncturists. These acupuncturists are blinded to the trial results and asked to rate whether the acupuncture provided was adequate to address the condition based on five aspects of treatment (the points selected, the total number of treatments, the number of times per week the patient was treated, the duration of each session and whether or not *de chi* was elicited). Unfortunately, this method proved very complex and the data were not interpretable (personal communication).

A second approach used by Molsberger and Bowing (1997) defines a minimally adequate acupuncture treatment as consisting of at least ten total treatments of at least fifteen minutes each and a description of the points used. Only sixteen of eighty-eight studies on musculoskeletal or neurological conditions met these minimal criteria.

A third approach has used textbooks from China, Japan and Korea (Birch 1997) to formulate criteria for treatment adequacy (Ezzo et al. 2000). This work tests the hypotheses that: six points per treatment are adequate but ten are even better, six total treatments are adequate but ten are even better, and that these parameters are associated with positive outcomes. The criteria for specific points used could not be set because these varied between textbooks.

When these hypotheses were tested, no association was observed between the number of points used and positive outcome, but a statistically significant association ($P<0.05$) was found between the total number of treatments given and a positive outcome, even when controlling for methodological quality of the trials. Virtually no trial that administered less than six acupuncture treatments achieved a positive outcome. Although these significant findings suggest association and not causation, the findings may be a starting point to examine dose–response relationships in pilot tests prior to conducting larger trials.

There is no consensus about how to assess treatment adequacy. In the Cochrane protocol for manual lymphatic drainage (MLD) (Howell et al. 2002) it is suggested that two MLD-certified therapists blinded to study results assign a wholistic score of 'adequate', 'inadequate' or 'not enough information to decide' to each of the treatment regimens based on their clinical experience. This simple method has been used in the acupuncture-point stimulation for chemotherapy-induced nausea and vomiting (Ezzo et al. in press) and has been found to attract high inter-rater agreement.

Initially, the Cochrane peer review disagreed with this approach, suggesting the use of explicit criteria for each treatment dimension such as number of treatments, duration of treatment session and frequency of treatments. It was explained that this method had been ruled out given Linde's lack of enthusiasm after having tried it. Ultimately, the Cochrane peer review accepted the wholistic scoring method.

Under-reporting is a common barrier to assessing treatment adequacy. Indeed, data on de chi are reported so infrequently in acupuncture trials that it cannot be meaningfully assessed (Ezzo et al. 2000). Similarly, so few treatment details are reported in massage trials (Haraldsson et al. 2004) that rather than assessing the treatments it is perhaps beneficial to report and discuss the under-reporting problem with hopes of influencing reporting practices in the future.

Treatment adequacy is particularly difficult to assess in mind–body therapies such as meditation. Although meditation is a self-administered therapy, unlike other self-administered therapies such as ingestible substances, compliance with meditation practice does not ensure treatment adequacy. Since compliance is not a good proxy for treatment adequacy, researchers have sought physiological measures that can serve as proxies. However, changes in heart rate or respiratory rate can be achieved by a variety of activities, even reading silently, and, therefore, cannot be used to assess treatment adequacy in meditation trials (Caspi and Burleson 2003). Treatment adequacy in CAM ingestible substances requires standardised samples containing active ingredient(s). The predominant limitation of existing botanical trials cited in systematic reviews is the lack of standardised samples.

Practitioner qualifications

Evaluating *efficacy* means testing an intervention under optimal conditions. This does not guarantee that the benefits of the intervention will carry over in the real world uses (*effectiveness*), but the efficacy principal does give an intervention the best opportunity to prove itself. Optimal conditions require not only adequate doses, but also excellent practitioners in practitioner-based modalities such as massage, acupuncture and chiropractic. Anyone who has visited more than one practitioner of the same modality knows that practitioners' skills vary widely. If an intervention is administered by a less than highly skilled practitioner the trial may be assessing effectiveness rather than efficacy.

Commentators have highlighted three dimensions that relate to practitioner quality: credentials, experience and hands-on proficiency (Eisenberg et al. 2002). Ter Riet et al. (1990) felt that the practitioner qualifications played such an important role in chronic-pain outcomes for acupuncture that they attempted to use practitioner credentials and practitioner experience as a proxy for adequacy of treatment. However, these details were so seldom reported that the reviewers could draw no conclusions. Haraldsson et al. (2004) noted the same under-reporting of practitioners' qualifications in a massage review.

The under-reporting of practitioner qualifications may reflect the lack of serious consideration given to this issue in trial planning. While this issue extends to all practitioner-based modalities, the issue is well illustrated by examples in massage research. Against a backdrop of trials that give no details of practitioner selection, some trials stand out for their conscientious consideration of practitioner selection. The multi-centre 'Relieving End-of-life Symptoms with Massage' (REST) study (work in progress at the time of writing) has hired only certified massage therapists with prior experience treating dying patients. Similarly, in a 'massage for low back pain' trial, Cherkin et al. (2003) required not only certification and prior experience treating low back pain, but also a 'hands-on working interview' in which researchers received a massage from each therapist prior to being hired.

In systematic reviews, the problem arises as to how massage trials which have made efforts to use highly skilled practitioners can be compared with trials where massage has been administered by massage students, chiropractic assistants with no formal massage training or nurses trained in massage only for the study but with no prior experience. Can these latter trials really be considered efficacy trials? At the simplest level, one might do a subgroup analysis comparing trials of more versus less qualified practitioners. However, this issue is far from resolved. Some suggest that the need for highly skilled practitioners varies from condition to condition. For example, some believe that nurses with no formal massage training other than for the purposes of the study are sufficient to administer very basic, formulaic massage to premature infants (Field et al. 1987). Presently, the vast majority of reviews are left to comment on the lack of reporting of practitioner selection criteria in the hope of both raising standards for reporting and, most importantly, raising standards of selection during planning of trials.

Cointerventions

CAM, by definition, is often an add-on treatment. Yet, it is often impossible in CAM systematic reviews to assess cointerventions because they have not been adequately documented in the clinical trials. Nevertheless, it remains that when a conventional treatment is universally and simultaneously used with CAM by a study population and that intervention becomes more effective over time, it can alter the relative benefit of the CAM treatment. In such cases, the impact of the cointervention must be considered.

For example, the 1998 National Institutes of Health (NIH) Consensus statement (Anonymous 1998) concluded that acupuncture was effective for chemotherapy-induced illness. However, the most recent (and most efficacious) generation of antiemetics (5-HT$_3$ inhibitors such as ondansetron and granisetron) was only just beginning to be widely used at the time of this statement. When the review of acupuncture for chemotherapy-induced nausea and vomiting began shortly after the NIH conference, there was a question as to whether these more highly efficacious antiemetics would change the relative contribution of acupuncture. Thus, the review needed to take into account the patients' use of antiemetics while receiving acupuncture treatment. Antiemetic regimens are determined based on the emetogenicity rating of the chemotherapy. A rating achieved through an oncologist assessing the chemotherapy, the emetogenicity ratings and the compliance with modern antiemetic guidelines. Trial investigators provided missing data and subgroup analysis was performed comparing modern and older antiemetics. The results showed that all acupuncture trials gave concomitant antiemetics, and the pooled acupuncture results showed a protective effect. However, no acupuncture trial had given antiemetics wholly consistent with current standards. The positive findings were a 'proof of principle' of acupuncture's effectiveness but could not answer whether acupuncture added benefit to modern antiemetics (Ezzo et al. in press).

Interpreting results

Generally by the time the review's conclusions are written, reviewers agree on data interpretation. However, such agreement is not always the case. In the 'acupuncture for chemotherapy-induced nausea and vomiting' review, one methodologist interpreted the results differently from the other participating methodologists. While one reviewer suggested that acupuncture may be beneficial for refractory patients, others argued no trials had explicitly assessed refractory patients. The point of the dissenting methodologist was that refractory patients were out of options, that acupuncture is safe and, based on the proof of principle from high-quality randomised trials, it may be beneficial. Reviewers spent an additional month consulting external experts – oncologists, oncology biostatisticians and epidemiologists – as well as discussing the issue internally. After much discussion, the decision was made to not suggest acupuncture for refractory patients but to suggest further trials need to be conducted (Ezzo et al. in press).

Safety

Safety, not just efficacy, needs to be addressed systematically. Safety data on CAM dietary supplements are particularly challenging due to their lack of government regulation in certain countries where there is high use such as the USA. As such, adverse-events documentation relies on self-initiated reporting, resulting in under-reporting. Incidence rates of adverse events, therefore, cannot be directly calculated for ingestible substances because the numerator (number of adverse events) is under-reported, and the denominator (number of persons using the substance) is extremely difficult if not impossible to estimate.

For safety to be evaluated in systematic reviews, assessments need to go beyond the clinical trials, which are notoriously small, and into other sources such as drug-interaction databases, population-based surveys and manufacturers' records. Cost, however, remains an obstacle. Some reviews have an explicit and transparent method for assessing adverse effects (Mulrow et al. 2000) although most lack this level of detail. Increasingly, CAM reviews at least cite contraindications and possible side effects even when they lack a search of adverse events.

Incidence rates of adverse events of practitioner-based modalities are easier to approximate because they can be assessed through large prospective studies of clinical practices with the consecutive patients providing the denominator. This method has been used in acupuncture (Ernst and White 2001, MacPherson et al. 2001), massage (Cassileth and Vickers 2004), and chiropractic (Cagnie et al. 2004, Haas et al. 2004). Systematic reviews of the prospective studies have also been done (Ernst and White 2001).

Summary

Systematic reviews are an evolving science and need to have the same methodological rigor as any other study design. In addition to the methodological issues that apply to all reviews, CAM systematic reviews often have to address additional methodological issues given the complexity of CAM interventions. CAM systematic reviews are particularly valuable not only for their summaries of the evidence but also for the way in which they provide valuable information to guide subsequent clinical research.

Note

Both authors contributed equally to this work.

Acknowledgements

Eric Manheimer was partially funded by grant number R24 AT001293 from the National Center for Complementary and Alternative Medicine (NCCAM). The contents of this article are solely the responsibility of the authors and do not necessarily represent the official views of the NCCAM or the National Institutes of Health.

References

Anonymous (1998) 'NIH Consensus Conference: acupuncture', *Journal of the American Medical Association*, 280 (17): 1518–24.

Atkins, D., Best, D., Briss, P. A., Eccles, M., Falck-Ytter, Y., Flottorp, S., Guyatt, G. H., Harbour, R. T., Haugh, M. C., Henry, D., Hill, S., Jaeschke, R., Leng, G., Liberati, A., Magrini, N., Mason, J., Middleton, P., Mrukowicz, J., O'Connell, D., Oxman, A. D., Phillips, B., Schunemann, H. J., Edejer, T. T., Varonen, H., Vist, G. E., Williams, J. W. and Zaza, S. (2004) 'Grading quality of evidence and strength of recommendations', *British Medical Journal*, 328 (7454): 1490.

Avenell, A., Handoll, H. H. and Grant, A. M. (2001) 'Lessons for search strategies from a systematic review in the Cochrane Library of nutritional supplementation trials in patients after hip fracture', *American Journal of Clinical Nutrition*, 73 (3): 505–10.

Bausell, R. B., Lao, L., Bergman, S., Lee, W. L. and Berman, B. M. (2005) 'Is acupuncture analgesia an expectancy effect? Preliminary evidence based on participants' perceived assignments in two placebo-controlled trials', *Evaluation and Health Professions*, 28 (1): 9–26.

Begg, C., Cho, M., Eastwood, S., Horton, R., Moher, D., Olkin, I., Pitkin, R., Rennie, D., Schulz, K. F., Simel, D. and Stroup, D. F. (1998) 'Improving the quality of reporting of randomized controlled trials: the CONSORT statement', *Revista Espanola de Salud Publica*, 72 (1): 5–11.

Berman, B. M., Lao, L., Langenberg, P., Lee, W. L., Gilpin, A. M. and Hochberg, M. C. (2004) 'Effectiveness of acupuncture as adjunctive therapy in osteoarthritis of the knee: a randomized, controlled trial', *Annals of Internal Medicine*, 141 (12): 901–10.

Bero, L. A. and Jadad, A. R. (1997) 'How consumers and policymakers can use systematic reviews for decision making', *Annals of Internal Medicine*, 127 (1): 37–42.

Birch, S. (1997) 'An Exploration with Proposed Solutions of the Problems and Issues in Conducting Clinical Research in Acupuncture', Ph.D. thesis, University of Exeter.

Cagnie, B., Vinck, E., Beernaert, A. and Cambier, D. (2004) 'How common are side effects of spinal manipulation and can these side effects be predicted?', Manual Therapy, 9 (3): 151–6.

Caspi, O. and Burleson, K. O. (2003) 'Methodological challenges in meditation research', Advances in Mind-Body Medicine, 21 (1): 4–11.

Cassileth, B. R. and Vickers, A. J. (2004) 'Massage therapy for symptom control: outcome study at a major cancer center', Journal of Pain and Symptom Management, 28 (3): 244–9.

Chalmers, I. (2001) 'Using systematic reviews and registers of ongoing trials for scientific and ethical trial design, monitoring, and reporting', in S. G. Davey and D. G. Altman (eds) Systematic Reviews in Health Care: Meta-Analysis in Context, London: BMJ Books, pp. 429–43.

Cherkin, D. C., Sherman, K. J., Deyo, R. A. and Shekelle, P. G. (2003) 'A review of the evidence for the effectiveness, safety, and cost of acupuncture, massage therapy, and spinal manipulation for back pain', Annals of Internal Medicine, 138 (11): 898–906.

The Cochrane Collaboration (2005) 'Cochrane Collaboration Policy on Commercial Sponsorship', Available online at <http://www.cochrane.org/docs/commercialsponsorship.htm> (accessed 2 February 2005).

Deeks, J. J., Higgins, J. P. T. and Altman, D. G. (2005) 'Analysing and presenting results', in J. P. T. Higgins and S. Green (eds) Cochrane Handbook for Systematic Reviews of Interventions 4.2.4 Section 8, Available online at <http://www.cochrane.org/resources/handbook/hbook.htm> (accessed 3 June 2005).

Diamond B. J., Johnson, S. K., Torsney, K., Morodan, J., Prokop, B. J., Davidek, D. and Kramer, P. (2003) 'Complementary and alternative medicines in the treatment of dementia: an evidence-based review', Drugs and Aging, 20 (13): 981–98.

Dickersin, K. and Manheimer, E. (1998) 'The Cochrane Collaboration: evaluation of health care and services using systematic reviews of the results of randomized controlled trials', Clinical Obstetrics and Gynecology, 41 (2): 315–31.

Dickersin, K., Scherer, R. and Lefebvre, C. (1994) 'Identifying relevant studies for systematic reviews', British Medical Journal, 309 (6964): 1286–91.

Egger, M., Juni, P., Bartlett, C., Holenstein, F. and Sterne, J. (2003) 'How important are comprehensive literature searches and the assessment of trial quality in systematic reviews? Empirical study', Health Technology Assessment, 7 (1): 1–76.

Eisenberg, D. M., Cohen, M. H., Hrbek, A., Grayzel, J., Van Rompay, M. I. and Cooper, R. A. (2002) 'Credentialing complementary and alternative medical providers', Annals of Internal Medicine, 137 (12): 965–73.

Ernst, E. and White, A. R. (2001) 'Prospective studies of the safety of acupuncture: a systematic review', The American Journal of Medicine, 110 (6): 481–5.

Ezzo, J., Berman, B., Hadhazy, V. A., Jadad, A. R., Lao, L. and Singh, B. B. (2000) 'Is acupuncture effective for the treatment of chronic pain? A systematic review', Pain, 86 (3): 217–25.

Ezzo, J., Hadhazy, V., Birch, S., Lao, L., Kaplan, G., Hochberg, M. and Berman, B. (2001) 'Acupuncture for osteoarthritis of the knee: a systematic review', Arthritis and Rheumatism, 44 (4): 819–25.

Ezzo J., Vickers A. J., Richardson, M. A., Allen, C., Dibble, S., Issell, B., Lao, L.,

Pearl, M., Ramirez, G., Roscoe, J., Shen, J., Shivnan, J., Streitberger, K., Treish, I. and Zhang, G. (2005) 'Acupuncture-point stimulation for chemotherapy-induced nausea and vomiting: a systematic review', *Journal of Clinical Oncology*, 23 (28): 7188–98.

Field, T., Scafidi, F. and Schanberg, S. (1987) 'Massage of preterm newborns to improve growth and development', *Paediatric Nursing*, 13 (6): 385–7.

Furlan, A. D., van Tulder, M. W., Cherkin, D. C., Tsukayama, H., Lao, L., Koes, B. W. and Berman, B. M. (2005) 'Acupuncture and dry-needling for low back pain', *Cochrane Database Systematic Review* Issue 1. Art. No.: CD001351.pub2. DOI: 10.1002/14651858.CD001351.pub2.

Haas, M., Goldberg, B., Aickin, M., Ganger, B. and Attwood, M. (2004) 'A practice-based study of patients with acute and chronic low back pain attending primary care and chiropractic physicians: two-week to 48-month follow-up', *Journal of Manipulative and Physiological Therapeutics*, 27 (3): 160–9.

Haraldsson, B. G., Gross, A. R., Goldsmith, C. H., Myers, C. D., Ezzo, J. M., Morien, A. and Peloso, P. (Cervical Overview Group) (2004) 'Massage for mechanical neck disorders', *(Protocol) Cochrane Database Systematic Review* Issue 3. Art. No.: CD004871. DOI: 10.1002/14651858.CD004871.pub2.

Higgins, J. P. T. and Green, S. (eds) *Cochrane Handbook for Systematic Reviews of Interventions*, 4.2.4. Available online at <http://www.cochrane.org/resources/handbook/hbook.htm> (accessed 31 March 2005).

Howell, D., Ezzo, J., Tuppo, K., Bily, L. and Johannson, K. (2002) 'Complete decongestive therapy for lymphedema following breast cancer treatment', *(Protocol) Cochrane Database Systematic Review*, Issue 1. Art. No.: CD003475. DOI: 10.1002/14651858.CD003475.

Jadad, A. R., Moore, R. A., Carroll, D., Jenkinson, C., Reynolds, D. J., Gavaghan, D. J. and McQuay, H. J. (1996) 'Assessing the quality of reports of randomized clinical trials: is blinding necessary?', *Controlled Clinical Trials*, 17: 1–12.

Jadad, A. R., Cook, D. J., Jones, A., Klassen, T. P., Tugwell, P., Moher, M. and Moher, D. (1998) 'Methodology and reports of systematic reviews and meta-analyses: a comparison of Cochrane reviews with articles published in paper-based journals', *Journal of the American Medical Association*, 280 (1): 278–80.

Juni, P., Altman, D. G. and Egger, M. (2001) 'Systematic reviews in health care: assessing the quality of controlled clinical trials', *British Medical Journal*, 323 (7303): 42–6.

Juni, P., Holenstein, F., Sterne, J., Bartlett, C. and Egger, M. (2002) 'Direction and impact of language bias in meta-analyses of controlled trials: empirical study', *International Journal of Epidemiology*, 31 (1): 115–23.

Knipschild, P. (1994) 'Systematic reviews: some examples', *British Medical Journal*, 309 (6986): 719–21.

Lao, L. (2005) 'Commentary on Sood et al: Cochrane systematic reviews in acupuncture: methodological diversity in database searching', *Journal of Alternative and Complementary Medicine*, 11 (4): 723–4.

Lehmann, H. P. and Goodman, S. N. (1995) 'Specifications for formalizing clinical significance', *Medical Decision Making*, 15: 424.

LeLorier, J., Gregoire, G., Benhaddad, A., Lapierre, J. and Derderian, F. (1997) 'Discrepancies between meta-analyses and subsequent large randomized, controlled trials', *New England Journal of Medicine*, 337 (8): 536–42.

Lewith, G. T., Walach, H. and Jonas, W. B. (2002) 'Balanced research strategies for complementary and alternative medicine', in G. T. Lewith, W. B. Jonas and H. Walach (eds) *Clinical Research in Complementary Therapies: Principles, Problems and Solutions*, Edinburgh: Churchill Livingstone.

Linde, K. and Willich, S. N. (2003) 'How objective are systematic reviews? Differences between reviews on complementary medicine', *Journal of the Royal Society of Medicine*, 96 (1): 17–22.

Linde, K., Jobst, K. and Panton, J. (1996) 'Acupuncture for chronic asthma', *Cochrane Database Systematic Reviews*, Issue 2.

Linde, K., Streng, A., Jurgens, S., Hoppe, A., Brinkhaus, B., Witt, C., Wagenpfeil, S., Pfaffenrath, V., Hammes, M. G., Weidenhammer, W., Willich, S. N. and Melchart, D. (2005) 'Acupuncture for patients with migraine: a randomized controlled trial', *Journal of the American Medical Association*, 293 (17): 2118–25.

Manheimer, E. and Berman, B. (2005) 'The Cochrane column: exploring, evaluating, and applying the results of systematic reviews of CAM therapies', *Explore: The Journal of Science and Healing*, 1 (3): 210–14.

Manheimer, E., White, A., Berman, B., Forys, K. and Ernst, E. (2005) 'Meta-analysis: acupuncture for low back pain', *Annals of Internal Medicine*, 142 (8): 651–63.

Manheimer, E., Ezzo, J., Hadhazy, V. and Berman, B. (in press) 'In a comparison of randomization and blinding of trial publications and investigator surveys, allocation concealment was under-reported', *Journal of Clinical Epidemiology*.

McCarney, R. W., Brinkhaus, B., Lasserson, T. J. and Linde, K. (2003) 'Acupuncture for chronic asthma', *The Cochrane Database of Systematic Reviews* Issue 3. Art. No.: CD000008. DOI: 10.1002/14651858.CD000008.pub2.

McNeely, M. L., Magee, D. J., Lees, A. W., Bagnall, K. M., Haykowsky, M. and Hanson, J. (2004) 'The addition of manual lymph drainage to compression therapy for breast cancer related lymphedema: a randomized controlled trial', *Breast Cancer Research Treatment*, 86 (2): 95–106.

MacPherson, H., White, A., Cummings, M., Jobst, K. A., Rose, K. and Niemtzow, R. C. (2002) 'Standards for reporting interventions in controlled trials of acupuncture: the STRICTA recommendations', *Journal of Alternative and Complementary Medicine*, 8 (1): 85–9.

MacPherson, H., Thomas, K., Walters, S. and Fitter, M. (2001) 'The York acupuncture safety study: prospective survey of 34 000 treatments by traditional acupuncturists', *British Medical Journal*, 323 (7311): 486–7.

Moher, D., Fortin, P., Jadad, A. R., Juni, P., Klassen, T., Le Lorier, J., Liberati, A., Linde, K. and Penna, A. (1996) 'Completeness of reporting of trials published in languages other than English: implications for conduct and reporting of systematic reviews', *Lancet*, 347 (8998): 363–6.

Moher, D., Pham, B., Klassen, T. P., Schulz, K. F., Berlin, J. A., Jadad, A. R. and Liberati, A. (2000) 'What contributions do languages other than English make on the results of meta-analyses?', *Journal of Clinical Epidemiology*, 53 (9): 964–72.

Moher, D., Pham, B., Lawson, M. L., and Klassen, T. P. (2003) 'The inclusion of reports of randomised trials published in languages other than English in systematic reviews', *Health Technology Assessment*, 7 (41): 1–90.

Moja, L. P., Telaro, E., D'Amico, R., Moschetti, I., Coe, L. and Liberati, A. (2005) 'Assessment of methodological quality of primary studies by systematic reviews:

results of the metaquality cross sectional study', *British Medical Journal*, 330 (7499): 1053.

Molsberger, A. and Bowing, G. (1997) 'Acupuncture for pain in locomotive disorders: critical analysis of clinical studies with respect to the quality of acupuncture in particular', *Schmerz*, 11 (1): 24–9.

Mulrow, C. D. (1987) 'The medical review article: state of the science', *Annals of Internal Medicine*, 106 (3): 485–8.

Mulrow, C., Lawrence, V., Jacobs, B. (2000) 'Milk thistle: effects on liver disease and cirrhosis and clinical adverse effects', *Evidence Report/Technology Assessment No. 21*, Rockville, Md.: Agency for Healthcare Research and Quality.

Murphy, L. S., Reinsch, S., Najm, W. I., Dickerson, V. M., Seffinger, M. A., Adams, A. and Mishra, S. I. (2003) 'Searching biomedical databases on complementary medicine: the use of controlled vocabulary among authors, indexers and investigators', *BMC Complementary Alternative Medicine*, 3: 3.

Paterson, C. and Dieppe, P. (2005) 'Characteristic and incidental (placebo) effects in complex interventions such as acupuncture', *British Medical Journal*, 330 (7501): 1202–5.

Patsopoulos, N. A., Analatos, A. A. and Ioannidis, J. P. (2005) 'Relative citation impact of various study designs in the health sciences', *Journal of the American Medical Association*, 293 (19): 2362–6.

Pilkington, K. and Richardson, J. (2004) 'Exploring the evidence: the challenges of searching for research on acupuncture', *Journal of Alternative and Complementary Medicine*, 10 (3): 587–90.

Pilkington, K., Boshnakova, A., Clarke, M. and Richardson, J. (2005) ' "No language restrictions" in database searches: what does this really mean?', *Journal of Alternative and Complementary Medicine*, 11 (1): 205–7.

Savoie, I., Helmer, D., Green, C. J. and Kazanjian, A. (2003) 'Beyond Medline: reducing bias through extended systematic review search', *International Journal of Technology Assessment in Health Care*, 19 (1): 168–78.

ter Riet, G., Kleijnen, J. and Knipschild, P. (1990) 'Acupuncture and chronic pain: a criteria-based meta-analysis', *Journal of Clinical Epidemiology*, 43 (11): 1191–9.

van Tulder, M. W., Cherkin, D., Berman, B., Lao, L. and Koes, B. W. (1999) 'Acupuncture for low back pain', *Cochrane Database Systematic Review*, 2, Chichester: John Wiley and Sons. 10.1002/14651858.CD001351.

van Tulder, M., Furlan, A., Bombardier, C. and Bouter, L. (2003) 'Updated method guidelines for systematic reviews in the Cochrane collaboration back review group', *Spine*, 28 (12): 1290–9.

Vickers, A., Goyal, N., Harland, R. and Rees, R. (1998) 'Do certain countries produce only positive results? A systematic review of controlled trials', *Controlled Clinical Trials*, 19 (2): 159–66.

Young, C. and Horton, R. (2005) 'Putting clinical trials into context', *Lancet*, 366 (9480): 107–8.

Chapter 3

Utilising existing data sets for CAM-consumption research

The case of cohort studies

David Sibbritt

Introduction

Health-related data sets resulting from cohort or longitudinal studies (studies where a group of people are followed in terms of their health experiences over many years) are abundant throughout the world. While the research aim and scope of such studies does not necessarily include CAM, some are concerned with CAM-related issues (for example, consultation with a CAM practitioner and the consumption of vitamin/mineral/herbal supplements). A focused analysis of CAM users is often neglected in these studies and, as such, the opportunity to explore a rich source of information on CAM use and CAM users often remains overlooked.

This chapter draws upon the experience of the author in conducting CAM-focused secondary data analysis (SDA) of cohort studies to help describe the advantages and disadvantages of analysing existing data sets with a view to CAM use and users. The chapter provides insight into the statistical issues that arise with such analysis and assumes a first-year-undergraduate level of statistical knowledge. Readers looking to explore basic statistics should consult more general texts in the field (for example, Bland 2000).

CAM use and CAM users: a brief literature review

There are a considerable number of studies in the literature that have reported information on CAM use and CAM users. Most relate to specific modalities (Norheim and Fonnebo 2000, Coulter et al. 2002, Cramer et al. 2003) or the treatment of patients with specific diseases or symptoms (Schafer et al. 2002, Keenan et al. 2003, Haetzman et al. 2003, Sibbritt et al. 2003, Mehrotra et al. 2004). However, for brevity, this literature review focuses upon only those studies that have reported CAM use – defined as a group of CAM modalities – amongst the general community. Such studies can be categorised into those designed with the primary research aim of eliciting information regarding CAM use and those where information regarding CAM use results from SDA of an existing study database.

In studies where the design is primarily guided by a focus on CAM consumption, findings have identified CAM users, in comparison to CAM non-users, as more likely to:

- be female (MacLennan et al. 1996, Thomas et al. 2001, Emslie et al. 2002, Shmueli and Shuval 2004, Al-Windi 2004, Lim et al. 2005);
- be aged between thirty-five and forty-nine years of age (Thomas et al. 2001, Emslie et al. 2002, Al-Windi 2004);
- have a higher income (Shmueli and Shuval 2004, Al-Windi 2004);
- have a higher level of education (Shmueli and Shuval 2004, Al-Windi 2004);
- reside in non-urban areas (MacLennan et al. 1996);
- be in full time employment (MacLennan et al. 1996, Thomas et al. 2001, Al-Windi 2004);
- have a poor health status (MacLennan et al. 1996, Al-Windi 2004). In addition, CAM users appear to employ CAM in conjunction with conventional health services (Emslie et al. 2002, Shmueli and Shuval 2004, Al-Windi 2004).

Although these studies highlight similar characteristics of CAM users, there is substantial variation in the prevalence of CAM use reported, ranging from between 6 per cent to 70 per cent. One factor influencing these findings relates to how CAM use is defined across the various studies. Some studies only consider consultation with a CAM practitioner as constituting CAM use (Adams et al. 2003b, Schmueli and Shuval 2004, Upchurch and Chyu 2005) while others also include use of self-prescribed CAM medications (MacLennan et al. 1996, Thomas et al. 2001, Wilkinson and Simpson 2001, Emslie et al. 2002). The number of CAM practitioners or CAM medications listed also varies greatly between the different studies. For example, the study by Barnes et al. (2004) includes twenty-seven types of CAM (ten types of provider-based CAM therapies and seventeen other CAM therapies for which the services of a practitioner are not necessary), while the study by Upchurch and Chyu (2005) includes twelve types of provider-based CAM therapies.

In addition to this CAM primary focused work has been a number of studies on CAM use based on SDA of existing study databases (Adams et al. 2003a or b, Sibbritt et al. 2003, Sibbritt et al. 2004, Steinsbekk et al. 2006). For example, many studies have analysed the National Health Interview Survey (NHIS) data conducted in the USA over a number of years (Kessler et al. 2001, Tindle et al. 2005, Upchurch and Chyu 2005). These studies report similar findings to those mentioned above, with higher CAM use reported among females, those with a higher income, a higher education, of mid-age and in poorer health. It is interesting to note that even though all these studies analyse NHIS data, longitudinal comparisons across the survey time periods have proved difficult due to changes in the wording of questions on CAM use, the sampling strategies and mode of administration (Tindle et al. 2005).

In terms of future directions for CAM use and user research, commentators have highlighted the need for longitudinal (or cohort) analyses to chart the trends in CAM consumption and the need for international comparative analyses to obtain a cross-cultural perspective to health and CAM (Adams et al. 2003a). As such writing highlights, there is a very real and significant role for the use of existing data sets and SDA in CAM-consumption research. Before exploring a number of benefits and challenges of such SDA it is first necessary to provide a brief overview of the SDA on CAM-consumption research that will serve as case studies and help illustrate relevant points later in the chapter.

Background to SDA on CAM consumption: the examples of WHA and HUNT

Recent years have seen the analysis on CAM-consumption data from two existing cohort studies: the Australian Longitudinal Survey of Women's Health (WHA) and the Nord-Trøndelag Health Study (HUNT). Both of these studies are longitudinal in design, are concerned with various health issues and have survey questions that elicit information about participants' CAM consumption. For both cohort studies, a sub-study team (including the author) has initiated and developed SDA for the purposes of examining CAM use and CAM users.

The WHA study was designed to investigate multiple factors affecting the health and well-being of women over a twenty-year period. Women in three age groups ('young' [eighteen to twenty-three], 'mid age' [forty-five to fifty] and 'older' [seventy to seventy-five]) were randomly selected from the national Medicare database, with over-representation of women living in rural and remote areas. The baseline survey was conducted in 1996 (n=14779 young, n=14099 mid age, and n=12939 older women).

The HUNT study is a population-based study conducted in the Nord-Trøndelag County, located in central Norway. The first phase of this study (HUNT 1) collected information on 74,599 persons aged twenty and older, and was primarily designed to cover four substudies (on hypertension, diabetes, lung diseases and quality of life). In the second phase (HUNT 2), there were 65,495 participants aged thirteen years and over. HUNT 2 used identical or similar questions and assessments on hypertension, diabetes and quality of life as in HUNT 1 but was much more comprehensive, with a wider age range and the collection of more data on each participant covering an extensive range of health-related topics.

It is important to note that while this chapter focuses upon cohort studies, not all SDA relating to CAM consumption is conducted on large cohort datasets. For example, an SDA of CAM use has been undertaken from an original survey designed to measure the supportive care needs of patients with cancer (Girgis et al. 2005). This survey contained questions in the 'background information' section asking patients about their use of a number of CAM modalities, allowing the creation of a 'CAM user' variable and subsequent modelling employing other variables measured in the survey instrument (Girgis et al. 2005).

Advantages of utilising existing cohort study data sets

Perhaps the greatest advantage afforded through analysis of an existing cohort data set for CAM consumption is simply its existence – this is particularly important given the potential difficulty in attracting research funding to undertake large-scale examination of CAM use. This may appear a less than ideal approach, but pre-existing data sets may in many circumstances constitute the only opportunity for CAM-consumption and CAM-user research. As well as benefits regarding funding, using pre-existing data sets also means data cleaning (checked for data errors, outliers, etc.) and a data dictionary (a database with question details and formats) will both have been completed prior to commencing the substudy – details and procedures that require much time and resources if undertaken from initial design.

There are also some useful statistical advantages in analysing cohort data sets. Typically, the data set will consist of a large sample of participants. This is obviously a design priority for the original researchers in terms of generating adequate statistical power to answer their specific research questions. As such, it is more than likely that there will also be sufficient statistical power to answer CAM-related research questions. These data sets will also tend to have information collected on many variables (including demographic, health-status and health-service-utilisation variables) allowing exploration of factors related to CAM consumption.

Finally, as study designs go, cohort studies are a highly regarded design, especially in comparison to cross-sectional studies (Christie et al. 1990). This is because they allow for the ability to consider longitudinal trends. Over time, different types of CAM users can be identified: those who consistently use CAM; those who consistently do not use CAM; and those who are intermittent users of CAM. Comparisons of these groups of CAM users and non-users can provide considerable insight into the knowledge about, and reasons for, CAM use over time (for more details see Sibbritt et al. 2005).

While studies on CAM use and users are beginning to attract some funding and attention (Wilder and Ernst 2003, Bensoussan and Lewith 2004) there remain many gaps in this field (Adams et al. 2003a). As this section has illustrated, SDA of pre-existing data sets is certainly one option that should, if possible, be considered by researchers looking to expand and enhance the investigation of CAM use and users. Nevertheless, pre-existing data sets and

SDA are not without their challenges and limitations. A number of these limitations, which should be adequately considered by any potential researcher contemplating SDA, are outlined and discussed below.

Limitations of utilising existing cohort-study data sets

A main limitation of using an existing data set to examine CAM use and CAM users is that the definition of CAM may not be ideal. For example, in the WHA questionnaire (conducted in 1996), the question relating to CAM was 'Have you consulted an alternative health practitioner (e.g. herbalist, chiropractor, naturopath, acupuncturist, etc.) in the last twelve months for your own health?' In this case, CAM use is defined as consultation with a CAM practitioner, but the definition excludes self-prescribed CAM use (such as vitamin and mineral supplements). Therefore, any prevalence of CAM use identified will be an underestimate of the true CAM use in the population. In addition, only a few examples of CAM practitioners are provided, and as such respondents may vary in the range of therapists they include under the heading of 'alternative practitioner'. It is not too surprising that these large cohort studies do not refine definition and nomenclature regarding CAM, after all there are often many competing areas for focus and CAM is not necessarily a primary consideration.

Another potential problem that may be encountered when attempting to analyse longitudinal trends in CAM consumption is a changing definition of CAM across different survey periods. For example, consider the wording of the questions used to determine CAM-user status for women in the young cohort of the WHA study. In time period 1 (1996), the definition of CAM-user status is defined by answers to the question: 'How many times have you consulted the following for your own health in the last 12 months? . . . [including, amongst a list of practitioners] an "alternative" health practitioner (e.g. chiropractor, naturopath, acupuncturist, herbalist etc)?' In time period 2 (1998), this definition of CAM-user status has changed somewhat and the question now reads: 'Have you consulted the following people for your own health in the last 12 months? . . . [including, amongst a list of practitioners] an "alternative" health practitioner (e.g. naturopath, acupuncturist, herbalist etc)?' Note that the question in time period 2 does not include chiropractor as an example of an alternative practitioner. In Australia, it has been shown that chiropractors are the most commonly consulted CAM-practitioner group (MacLennan et al. 2002). Given this context, a number of important questions are raised: How important is it that chiropractor was omitted from the example of CAM practitioners in time period 2? Will subjects consider chiropractors to be alternative health practitioners if they are not included in the examples list? If there is a decline in the number of subjects who indicate that they consulted a CAM practitioner, is it possible to know if there genuinely was a decline in CAM-practitioner consultation or is the decline due to subjects not considering chiropractors as being alternative health practitioners? In this particular study the change in definition was considered significant enough to preclude comparisons across the two time periods.

Using an existing data set has another disadvantage in that the reference population may be restricted by the study design; the population to whom the results can be generalised may be a subset of the community. For example, the WHA study was conducted only on women in certain age groups (eighteen to twenty-three, forty-five to fifty and seventy to seventy-five), who could speak/read English. In the case of the HUNT study, the population of Nord-Trøndelag County is in many respects a representative sample of the wider Norwegian population with regard to geography, economy, industry, sources of income, age distribution, morbidity and mortality. However, the county lacks a large city, and the level of education and income are somewhat lower than the national average. Nevertheless, it should be noted that these studies do provide some of the largest CAM-consumption data and analyses in the world (Adams et al. 2003b) and as explained earlier, the issue of sample size can in itself be considered a major benefit of conducting such SDA for CAM consumption.

Statistical analysis: issues and challenges

In this section I wish to discuss a number of statistical issues requiring consideration when conducting SDA. First, the analysis undertaken will depend on the number of time periods being analysed (for example, one time period, two time periods, three or more time periods). Second, it is necessary to be aware of the effect of missing data on study results and also several other minor issues are also worth highlighting (such as accounting for over-sampling, adjusting the level of statistical significance (P value) if the sample size is large, and how to handle the non-normality of distributions). Each of these issues is explored in turn in more detail below.

Analysing data over one, two or more time periods

One time point

The analysis of data at one point in time is straightforward and shall not be discussed in detail here. If a binary outcome variable does exist (for example, CAM user = yes or no), a 'profile' of CAM users can be developed by conducting two-way comparisons of CAM-user status against any number of predictor variables (such as gender, education, disease, etc.) using chi-square or t-test analyses (see Adams et al. 2003b). In addition, it is also possible to develop a multivariate model for identifying the important factors associated with CAM use via logistic regression (see McLennan et al. 2002).

Two time points

Analysis becomes more interesting when data collection incorporates multiple time points. For example, consider the situation when a binary outcome variable (for example, CAM user = yes or no) is measured on two occasions. One research gap that could be addressed from such a study design would be to determine if the proportion of CAM users is the same at Time 1 and Time 2.

The problem with comparing the proportion of CAM users over two time periods is that some important information may be overlooked. This was highlighted in Sibbritt et al. (2004) where it was shown that the percentage of CAM users at Time 1 was 28 per cent and this increased to 29 per cent at Time 2 (three years later). This tells us that across time the overall percentage of CAM users appears to be reasonably stable. However, what these figures 'hide' is the fact that 1,058 CAM users in Time 1 no longer used CAM in Time 2 and 1,146 CAM non-users in Time 1 became CAM users in Time 2. In a longitudinal analysis, where subjects' information is linked across time periods, it is these people who change their use of CAM over time that are probably more interesting than those who maintain the use or non-use of CAM over time. In line with this focus, the interesting questions now become: Why would subjects who used CAM in Time 1 choose not to use it in Time 2? Conversely, why would subjects who did not use CAM in Time 1 choose to use it in Time 2?

One approach to identifying the factors associated with change in CAM use that has been explored by myself and colleagues (Sibbritt et al. 2004) has been to construct two outcome measures to reflect the change in CAM-user status. Those subjects who were not CAM users in Time 1 but were identified as CAM users in Time 2 were defined as *CAM adopters*. Those subjects who were CAM users in Time 1 but not in Time 2 were defined as *CAM relinquishers*. Logistic regression was then applied to determine a model for identifying the factors associated with the adoption and relinquishment of CAM.

It is important to note that when applying logistic regressions in this manner, the analyses will be conducted on a subset of the larger data set. For example, following the example above, any modeling of CAM adopters would only consider those subjects who *do not* use CAM at Time 1. In addition, the CAM adopters are those who use CAM at Time 2 and do not use CAM at Time 1, and they would be compared to those subjects who do not use CAM at Time 2. Similarly, the CAM relinquisher modelling would be conducted only on those subjects who *do* use CAM at Time 1. The predictors used in such models would be representations of the change in factors over the two time periods. To explain, if area of residence (urban or rural) was a factor under consideration, then the representation of this factor used in the logistic regression model would be a variable with four levels: remained urban, moved from urban to non-urban, moved from non-urban to urban, remained non-urban (see Sibbritt et al. 2004).

A more sophisticated approach could be to use generalized estimating equations (GEE) analysis or random coefficient analysis. For both of these methods, there is no need to construct the CAM-adopter or CAM-relinquisher outcome variables as outlined above. These two methods can provide analysis of the changes or non-changes in CAM-user status over time using the one outcome variable (CAM user = yes or no). However, it is difficult for non-statisticians to understand the theory underlying these methods and thus it is difficult to correctly apply them to the data. For those interested, Twisk (2003) provides a good description of these longitudinal data-analysis methods.

More than two time points

The analysis of CAM use over three or more time periods presents further difficulty and complication. This is due to the number of possible combinations of CAM-user status a subject can be allocated (a status which increases by a factor of two for each additional time period being analysed). For example, Table 3.1 below shows that for three time periods, there are eight different combinations for CAM users. For four times periods, there would be sixteen different combinations, and so on.

This is a situation facing the WHA CAM substudy team with regard to the analysis of data from the WHA study, which now has collected health information on women over three time periods. The two sophisticated methods mentioned in the previous section (GEE analysis and random coefficient analysis) can both be applied when information is collected on more than two occasions, and these two methods may well prove to be the best approach to analysing CAM use and CAM users over three or more time periods. However, there may be a more straightforward solution.

With only three time points, there are five possible types of CAM users: consistent users, consistent non-users, CAM adopters, CAM relinquishers and intermittent users. *Consistent users* are those subjects who are CAM

Table 3.1 The possible combinations of CAM user status when measured over three time periods

Time 1	Time 2	Time 3
CAM user = No	CAM user = No	CAM user = No
CAM user = No	CAM user = No	CAM user = Yes
CAM user = No	CAM user = Yes	CAM user = No
CAM user = No	CAM user = Yes	CAM user = Yes
CAM user = Yes	CAM user = No	CAM user = No
CAM user = Yes	CAM user = No	CAM user = Yes
CAM user = Yes	CAM user = Yes	CAM user = No
CAM user = Yes	CAM user = Yes	CAM user = Yes

users at each time period, while *consistent non-users* are those subjects who are not CAM users at each time period. *CAM adopters* are those subjects who adopt CAM at Time 2 (and maintain their CAM use at Time 3) or adopt CAM at Time 3. *CAM relinquishers* are those subjects who relinquish CAM at Time 2 (and continue to not use CAM at Time 3) or relinquish CAM at Time 3. *Intermittent users* are those subjects who alternate their CAM use over the three time periods (user/non-user/user or non-user/user/non-user). Note that an assumption is made that the two different types of intermittent use of CAM can be treated as being equal with respect to the predictor variables in question. This approach to categorising CAM users over time is only useful for reporting prevalence (the percentage of subjects in each category) or conducting simple bivariate analyses (such as chi-square testing the association between CAM user status and a particular characteristic). It would not be practical to attempt to determine a statistical model to predict the factors associated with CAM status when it is defined by five categories – the interpretation would be extremely difficult. One solution would be to divide the analyses into two separate analyses, along the lines of that discussed in the previous section of this chapter. In both analyses, a polytomous logistic regression model (a logistic regression model for an outcome variable with more than two levels) could be generated for a CAM-user status-outcome variable with three levels along with various predictor variables. The outcome variables would be: (1) consistent CAM users, CAM relinquishers, intermittent users; and (2) consistent CAM non-users, CAM adopters, intermittent users.

As the number of possible combinations of CAM-user status increases (more time periods), some of these combinations will have very few subjects. For example, the number of consistent CAM users over five time periods may be extremely low and it may be necessary to define a consistent CAM user as those who use CAM over four or five time periods. It would not be ideal to define consistent CAM users in such a way, but if there are very few subjects who use CAM in all five time periods, then there may be insufficient statistical power to detect statistically significant relationships with this variable. Such decisions are ultimately study specific.

As with the case of two time periods, when there are three or more time periods under investigation, both GEE analysis or random coefficient analysis are appropriate. Given the problem of having too many possible combinations of CAM users, it is probably preferable to use one of these two modelling approaches.

Missing data

Another difficulty in analysing pre-existing data sets for CAM use and CAM users occurs when there is missing data (where there exist values of variables within a data set which are not known). Missing data can occur for a variety of reasons, namely missing completely at random (MCAR), missing at random (MAR), or missing not at random (MNAR). The effect that missing data has on the results depends on the reason why the data was missing. With regard to MCAR, the missingness of a variable is not related to that variable or to any other variable measured. For example, a respondent may have accidentally skipped a page of the questionnaire when responding. With MCAR, their missingness does not bias the results in favour of one group or the other. In practice, MCAR rarely occurs. It is more common that missingness is related to some variable that has been measured, but not to the outcome variable (MAR). An example of this is a question that attempts to elicit information on participants' personal income, which may be considered a sensitive question that participants may be reluctant to answer. Typically, data that are MCAR or MAR can be ignored because there are techniques that can be employed to 'fill in the gaps' (to impute the missing values). However, it is not possible to ignore data that are MNAR as they are missing because of the outcome variable. An example of MNAR is when participants drop out of a study concerning vision in the elderly because failing vision prevented them from reading and answering the questionnaire. (For more details on missing data see Verbeke and Molenberghs 2000, Diggle et al. 2002, Little and Rubin 2002.)

In relation to CAM, it is highly unlikely that data would be MNAR. Therefore, it is safe to assume that data relating to CAM would either be MCAR and MAR. There are several types of approaches used for dealing with missing data, but I will only consider the two most common approaches: complete case analysis and imputation methods. Complete case analysis is the simplest approach to handling missing data because all individuals with missing data are removed. The problem with this approach is that if the missing data is not random among certain groups within the study, then it may introduce a bias. Note that this method is the default in most statistical software. Under imputation, the missing values are replaced by some imputed value from the data, allowing for standard statistical analyses to be conducted. There are numerous imputation methods ranging from simple approaches such as mean imputation to more advanced multiple imputation. Details about the various imputation methods and their associated advantages and disadvantages can be found in Little and Rubin (2002).

Given that the focus of the bulk of this chapter is longitudinal CAM data it is useful to concentrate on some of the imputation methods that are more commonly used on such data. The simplest longitudinal imputation method is called the 'last value carried forward' method. Here, a missing value for a variable at a particular time point is replaced by the value for that individual's variable from the previous time point (the value is carried forward to the next time point). An alternative longitudinal imputation method is called the 'linear interpolation' method. Here, a missing value for a variable at a particular time point is replaced by a value obtained from a linear regression equation based on the non-missing values for that individual's variable from all other time points (Twisk 2003).

The multiple imputation method is the most sophisticated method for the imputation of missing data. Multiple imputation is a technique in which missing values for a variable are predicted (or imputed) using values from other variables. The missing values are replaced by the imputed values, resulting in a complete data set called an 'imputed data set'. This process is performed multiple times, producing multiple imputed data sets. With an imputed data set, a standard statistical analysis is then carried out on each imputed data set, producing multiple analysis results. These analysis results are then combined to produce one overall analysis. A good reference for multiple imputation is Rubin and Schenker (1991).

The important aspect of missing data that needs to be considered is what percentage of values is missing for a particular variable. A conservative 'rule of thumb' is to not impute values for a variable if more than 10 per cent of its values are missing. Similarly, complete case analysis should not be performed if more than 10 per cent of values are missing, as this would mean that information on 10 per cent of all participants would be ignored in the analyses. If a variable has more than 10 per cent missing values, then it should not be considered for analyses. My advice would be to even think carefully about variables that have between 5 and 10 per cent missing values. Note, that the participants who have missing values for one variable may not be the same ones who have missing values for another variable. So, if there are many variables under consideration the complete case analysis approach may result in a considerable number of participants' information being discarded.

If faced with a small data set, it is probably best to account for missing data using multiple imputation or the use of a GEE or random coefficient analysis, which can both produce models on data sets containing missing values. Fortunately, the cohort studies that I have been associated with have very large numbers of participants. Thus, in the CAM research that I have conducted using SDA of these cohort studies, I have only used complete case analyses. This decision was based on the fact that even after excluding information of participants with missing data a large number of participants remained and the assumption that the participants with missing information were not dissimilar to the participants with non-missing cases. However, as the number of time points increase, the need for GEE analysis or random coefficient analysis also increases, (almost) avoiding the decision about the appropriate method for handling missing data.

Other issues

In this section I wish to discuss two minor statistical issues that arise when the data set is based on a large sample size; adjusting the P value to define statistical significance and non-normality of distributions.

When analysing large data sets (for example, n>1,000), researchers may be surprised to find that many variables are associated with CAM – based on the typical P value of 0.05. In fact, if the sample size is very large (such as n>10,000) nearly all variables will be associated with CAM. If this occurs, does this mean that nearly all variables *are* associated with CAM? Probably not. The reason why is because significance levels obtained from statistical tests are determined from the standard error. The standard error is mostly dependent on sample size, such that with very large sample sizes, even negligible differences attain statistical significance (Glymour et al. 1997). In order to overcome this problem the level of statistical significance should be reduced. In this situation, a P value of 0.005 can be used (the results of a statistical test is considered to be statistically significant if P<0.005).

One of the assumptions of all parametric statistical tests (such as t-test, analysis of variance, linear regression) is that continuous variables are normally distributed. If this assumption is violated, then typically the offending variable would be transformed in some manner (for example, natural log transformation) or the particular parametric test would be discarded and replaced with an equivalent non-parametric test. The problem with transforming a variable is that interpretation of results becomes more difficult. For example, it is easier to deal with a variable *years of education* rather than the *square root of years of education*. As for non-parametric tests, they are more conservative than parametric tests, such that a statistically significant association that is detected between variables by a parametric test, may not be detected by a non-parametric test – although this is of lesser concern as the sample size increases. When faced with non-normal continuous variables, researchers could do worse than to take the view of Armitage and Berry (1987), who consider it appropriate and safe to still employ parametric tests when the sample size is large and regardless of the distribution of continuous variables.

Conclusion

Many health-related data sets, both cross-sectional and longitudinal, do exist around the world. Usually the study investigators are open to collaboration, especially if the potential collaborator is providing some additional expertise, such as knowledge of CAM. Conducting secondary data analyses are relatively easy, can expose early stage investigators to experienced researchers already involved in the study and can lead to additional analyses. For example, by analysing the WHA data with a focus on CAM use, the WHA CAM substudy team have been included in ongoing discussion regarding future surveys of the WHA cohorts, helping to refine the survey questions and thereby allowing the design of more interesting and pertinent CAM use and user research.

The statistical analyses of pre-existing data sets provide one interesting path to develop the CAM-user and CAM-consumption research field. Nevertheless, as this chapter suggests, such secondary analysis is not without its own particular difficulties. The definition of CAM users may not be ideal, the definition of CAM users may change over time when the study data is generated from a cohort, and the reference population may be restrictive. However, the advantages outweigh the disadvantages in that the data set exists, it may be void of difficulties associated with data collection, and most data errors are typically cleaned. As such, researchers can utilise the possible resource of SDA to help advance CAM-consumption research and to address a broad range of related questions regarding users, nature of use and patterns of use over time.

References

Adams, J., Easthope, G. and Sibbritt, D. (2003a) 'Exploring the relationship between women's health and the use of complementary and alternative medicine', *Complementary Therapies in Medicine*, 11 (3): 156–8.

Adams, J., Sibbritt, D., Easthope, G. and Young, A. (2003b) 'The profile of women who consult an alternative health practitioner in Australia', *Medical Journal of Australia*, 179 (6): 297–300.

Al-Windi, A. (2004) 'Determinants of complementary alternative medicine (CAM) use', *Complementary Therapies in Medicine*, 12 (2–3): 99–111.

Armitage, P. and Berry, G. (1987) *Statistical Methods in Medical Research*, Oxford: Blackwell.

Barnes, P., Powell-Griner, E., McFann, K. and Nahin, R. L. (2004) 'Complementary and alternative medicine use among adults: United States, 2002', *Advance Data*, 27 (343): 1–19.

Bensoussan, A. and Lewith, G. T. (2004) 'Complementary medicine research in Australia: a strategy for the future', *Medical Journal of Australia*, 81 (6): 331–3.

Bland, M. (2000) *An Introduction to Medical Statistics*, Oxford: Oxford University Press.

Chan, J. M., Elkin, E. P., Silva, S. J., Broering, J. M., Latini, D. M. and Carroll, P. R. (2005) 'Total and specific complementary and alternative medicine use in a large cohort of men with prostate cancer', *Urology*, 66 (6): 1223–8.

Christie, D., Gordon, I. and Heller, R. (1990) *Epidemiology: An Introductory Text for Medical and other Health Science Students*, Kensington: New South Wales University Press.

Coulter, I. D., Hurwitz, E. L., Adams, A. H., Genovese, B. J., Hays, R. and Shekelle, P. G. (2002) 'Patients using chiropractors in North America: who are they, and why are they in chiropractic care?', *Spine*, 27 (3): 291–7.

Cramer, E. H., Jones, P., Keenan, N. L. and Thompson, B. L. (2003) 'Is naturopathy as effective as conventional therapy for treatment of menopausal symptoms?', *The Journal of Alternative and Complementary Medicine*, 9 (4): 529–38.

Diggle, P. J., Heagerty, P. J., Liang, K., Zeger, S. L. (2002) *Analysis of Longitudinal Data*, Oxford: Oxford University Press.

Eisenberg, D. M., Davis, R. B., Ettner, S. L., Appel, S. M., Wilkey, S., Van Rompay,

M. I. and Kessler, R. C. (1998) 'Trends in alternative medicine use in the United States, 1990–1997: results of a follow-up national survey', *Journal of the American Medical Association*, 280 (18): 1569–75.

Emslie, M. J., Campbell, M. K. and Walker, K. A. (2002) 'Changes in public awareness of, attitudes to, and use of complementary therapy in North East Scotland: surveys in 1993 and 1999', *Complementary Therapies in Medicine*, 10 (3): 148–53.

Fouladbakhsh, J. M., Stommel, M., Given, B. A. and Given, C. W. (2005) 'Predictors of use of complementary and alternative therapies among patients with cancer', *Oncology Nursing Forum*, 32 (6): 1115–22.

Girgis, A., Adams, J. and Sibbritt, D. (2005) 'The use of complementary and alternative therapies by patients with cancer', *Oncology Research*, 15 (15): 281–289.

Glymour, C., Madigan, D., Pregibon, D. and Smyth, P. (1997) 'Statistical themes and lessons for data mining', *Data Mining and Knowledge Discovery*, 1 (1): 11–28.

Haetzman, M., Elliott, A. M., Smith, B. H. and Hannaford, P. (2003) 'Chronic pain and the use of conventional and alternative therapy', *Family Practice*, 20 (2): 147–54.

Hollyer, T., Boon, H., Georgousis, A., Smith, M. and Einarson, A. (2002) 'The use of CAM by women suffering from nausea and vomiting during pregnancy', *BMC Complementary and Alternative Medicine*, 2: 5–8.

Keenan, N. L., Fugh-Berman, M. S., Browne, D., Kaczmarczyk, J. and Hunter, C. (2003) 'Severity of menopausal symptoms and use of both conventional and complementary/alternative therapies', *Menopause*, 10 (6): 491–3.

Kessler, R. C., Davis, R. B., Foster, D. F., Van Rompay, M. I., Walters, E. E., Wilkey, S. A., Kaptchuk, T. J. and Eisenberg, D. M. (2001) 'Long-term trends in the use of complementary and alternative medicine therapies in the United States', *Annals of Internal Medicine*, 35 (4): 262–8.

Lim, M. K., Sadarangani, P., Chan, H. L. and Heng, J. Y. (2005) 'Complementary and alternative medicine use in multiracial Singapore', *Complementary Therapies in Medicine*, 13 (1): 16–24.

Little, R. J. A. and Rubin, D. B. (2002) *Statistical Analysis with Missing Data*, Hoboken, NJ: John Wiley and Sons.

McKay, D. J., Bentley, J. R. and Grimshaw, R. N. (2005) 'Complementary and alternative medicine in gynaecologic oncology', *Journal of Obstetrics and Gynaecology Canada*, 27 (6): 562–8.

MacLennan, A. H., Wilson, D. and Taylor, A. (1996) 'Prevalence and cost of alternative medicine in Australia', *Lancet*, 347 (9001): 569–73.

—— (2002) 'The escalating cost and prevalence of alternative medicine', Preventive Medicine, 35 (2): 166–73.

Mehrotra, R., Bajaj, S. and Kumar, D. (2004) 'Use of complementary and alternative medicine by patients with diabetes mellitus', *National Medical Journal of India*, 17 (5): 243–5.

Norheim, A. J. and Fonnebo, V. (2000) 'A survey of acupuncture patients: results from a questionnaire among a random sample in the general population in Norway', *Complementary Therapies in Medicine*, 8 (3): 187–92.

Rubin, D. B. and Schenker, N. (1991) 'Multiple imputation in health-care databases: an overview and some applications', *Statistics in Medicine*, 10 (4): 585–98.

Schafer, T., Riehle, A., Wichmann, H. and Ring, J. (2002) 'Alternative medicine in allergies: prevalence, patterns of use, and cost', *Allergy*, 57 (8): 694–700.

Shmueli, A. and Shuval, J. (2004) 'Use of complementary and alternative medicine in Israel: 2000 vs. 1993', *Israel Medical Association Journal*, 6: 3–8.

Sibbritt, D., Adams, J., Easthope, G. and Young, A. (2003) 'Complementary and Alternative Medicine (CAM) use among elderly Australian women who have cancer', *Supportive Care in Cancer*, 11 (8): 548–50.

Sibbritt, D., Adams, J. and Young, A. (2004) 'A longitudinal analysis of mid-aged women's use of complementary and alternative medicine (CAM) in Australia, 1996–1998', *Women and Health*, 40 (4): 41–56.

Steinsbekk, A., Adams, J., Sibbritt, D., Johnsen, R., Jacobsen, G. and Holmen, J. (2006) 'Socio-demographic characteristics and health perceptions among male and female CAM users in a Norwegian total population study (HUNT 2)', Internal Report, University of Newcastle, Australia.

Thomas, K., Nicholl, J. and Coleman, P. (2001) 'Use and expenditure on complementary medicine in England: a population based survey', *Complementary Therapies in Medicine*, 9 (1): 2–11.

Tindle, H. A., Davis, R. B., Phillips, R. S. and Eisenberg, D. M. (2005) 'Trends in use of complementary and alternative medicine by US adults: 1997–2002', *Alternative Therapies*, 11 (1): 42–9.

Twisk, J. (2003) *Applied Longitudinal Data Analysis for Epidemiology: A Practical Guide*, Cambridge: Cambridge University Press.

Upchurch, D. M. and Chyu, L. (2005) 'Use of complementary and alternative medicine among American women', *Women's Health Issues*, 15 (1): 5–13.

Verbeke, G. and Molenberghs, G. (2000) *Linear Mixed Models for Longitudinal Data*, New York: Springer-Verlag.

Wang, S. M., DeZinno, P., Fermo, L., William, K., Caldwell-Andrews, A. A., Bravemen, F. and Kain, Z. N. (2005) 'Complementary and alternative medicine for low-back pain in pregnancy: a cross-sectional survey', *Journal of Alternative and Complementary Medicine*, 11 (3): 459–64.

Wilder, B. and Ernst, E. (2003) 'CAM research funding in the UK: surveys of medical charities in 1999 and 2002', *Complementary Therapies in Medicine*, 11 (3): 165–7.

Wilkinson, J. and Simpson, M. (2001) 'High use of complementary therapies in a New South Wales rural community', *Australian Journal of Rural Health*, 9 (4): 166–71.

Chapter 4

Towards the application of RCTs for CAM

Methodological challenges

Marie Pirotta

Introduction

> Today RCTs are quite unequivocally associated with medicine, as the method of choice – the 'gold standard' – for evaluating the effectiveness of different health care treatments . . . It is difficult to arrive at knowledge in any other way except by controlling the wayward influences of chance. Once the operations of chance have been recognised, ways of knowing can never be the same again, chance . . . must be put firmly in its place.
>
> (Oakley 2000: 145 and 160)

Ideally, medicines should be subjected to rigorous research to establish effectiveness and safety – a point that applies to all medicines whether CAM or conventional (Angell and Jerome 1998). Nevertheless, many treatments have become established in practice without such a research base, such as bed rest for acute back pain (Allen et al. 1999), the use of lactobacillus probiotic to prevent vulvovaginal candidiasis after antibiotics (Pirotta et al. 2004) and the use of valerian for anxiety or insomnia (Jacobs et al. 2005). It is imperative that the research community work towards the goal of providing an evidence base for more medicines and treatments to enable consumers and health practitioners to make informed and safe choices about health care.

RCTs are acknowledged as the 'gold standard' for attributing cause and effect (i.e., to test whether an intervention truly is effective). RCTs have a relatively short history in clinical medicine. It has taken hundreds of years for orthodox medicine to accept evidence from research as a crucial underpinning of medical practice with ineffective and dangerous medical mainstays such as blood-letting remaining in vogue until the nineteenth century (Porter 1997). Around this time, the concept of clinical trials began to evolve, yet the crucial principle of random allocation of patients in trials was only first employed in 1948 to test spectinomycin for the treatment of tuberculosis (Doll 1998).

In brief, RCTs are designed specifically to test a therapy by comparing two (or more) experimental treatment groups. The rigour of the method is achieved by striving to ensure that the only difference between these groups is the therapy being tested. RCTs seek to minimise sources of bias, which could have an impact on the trial. The beauty of RCTs is that by randomly allocating participants into treatment groups, all known, and more importantly unknown, confounders should be distributed equally among groups so long as the sample size is adequate. A confounder is a factor, such as age or smoking, which may influence the outcome of the participants in the trial, yet may not be equally present in the treatment groups. The confounder may therefore account for part of the difference in outcomes, while not being part of the intervention tested.

When a research question is focused on the efficacy of a particular therapy, the RCT is the most rigorous method of choice, and in these circumstances researchers should aim to use this method wherever practical and ethical to do so (Levin et al. 1997). A hierarchy of evidence has been outlined with RCTs acknowledged as setting the highest standard of evidence with which to assess a therapy or treatment (Finkelstein and Rao 2005). However, there are obviously other research approaches and methods applicable to the study of health and health care, each with a distinct set of limitations and strengths. The choice of research method should ultimately be dictated by its suitability to answer or address the specific research question posed, while minimising bias (Vickers et al. 1997). For some research questions (for example, the types of practices used for certain conditions or how many patients are currently using a particular CAM [Vickers 1998, Nahin and Straus 2001]) research methods other than the RCT, such as surveys, qualitative research or observational studies may prove more appropriate and useful. A combination of qualitative and quantitative approaches may be best for other research questions, such as when evaluating the structures and processes of a complex health system (Verhoef et al. 2005).

The increasing popularity of CAM amongst patients (Eisenberg et al. 1993, Begbie et al. 1996, Ernst 2000, Gardiner and Wornham 2000, Harris and Rees 2000, MacLennan et al. 2002, Barnes et al. 2004) and a range of medical practitioners (Berman et al. 1995, White et al. 1997, Dobson 2003, Thomas et al. 2003, Cohen et al. 2005) has brought the lack of evidence base for CAM regarding efficacy and safety into focus, making CAM a legitimate area for research including the application of RCT methodology. Indeed, the role and development of RCTs for CAM is currently at a critical stage, and this chapter explores some issues that arise from the application of RCT methods to CAM research. However, prior to outlining these challenges and issues in more depth, it is first necessary to briefly explain 'the state of play' of RCTs in relation to CAM.

RCT method and CAM research: the state of play

Finally, after decades of being ignored or ridiculed by orthodox researchers and doctors, and with limited research being performed by enthusiasts with little training in research or funding, CAM research is now being accepted, indeed encouraged by both conventional and CAM practitioners (Kerr 1996, Angell and Jerome 1998, Fontanarosa and Lundberg 1998, Anonymous 2000, Chen and Ma 2001, Ernst 2001a, McCarthy 2002, Baldwin 2003). CAM RCTs currently range from designs typical of a pharmaceutical drug trial to complex designs that enable an entire system to be tested in its natural surrounds with highly individualised diagnosis and treatment (Nahin and Straus 2001, Verhoef et al. 2005).

Unfortunately, much of the early CAM RCT research was methodologically weak, leading to unreliable results that were unlikely to be published in reputable journals. For example, in 1995 the then entitled US National Institute of Health (NIH) Office of Alternative Medicine set itself the task of developing evidence-based clinical practice guidelines for CAM. One reason why this task was abandoned was a paucity of well-designed trials to inform such guidelines (Woolf et al. 1997). Likewise, a review of placebo-controlled homoeopathy trials identified two-thirds of the 186 trials as methodologically poor (Linde et al. 1997), and a review of acupuncture trials found that most had too small a sample size and were methodologically weak (Linde et al. 2001a).

To a large degree, the previous lack of methodological rigour in CAM RCT research may be understood as due to a difference in paradigms. Conventional medicine seeks to understand health and disease by reducing elements to their smallest parts (for example, focusing upon the roles of proteins, receptors or genes). In contrast, CAM approaches tend to be holistic, seeing the patient as a whole and as influenced by the environment and an inner spiritual domain. The RCT has developed from and is deeply embedded in the reductionist biomedical world and some have questioned or even rejected the suitability of this method for assessing the effectiveness of complementary systems of health care (Thompson 2004).

Indeed, it is important to acknowledge that there are aspects of complementary therapies that make the application of RCT methodology a special challenge. However, an expert panel convened by the US NIH pronounced no unique barriers to RCT CAM research on epistemological grounds (Levin et al. 1997) and many experts in the field have proposed the design of rigorous CAM trials that potentially satisfy both conventional and CAM proponents (Hensley and Gibson 1998, Nahin and Straus 2001, Ernst 2003).

This does not mean that the application of RCTs for investigating CAM is always a straightforward or simple matter. On the contrary, as this chapter will illustrate, there are a number of key issues that face the development of RCTs for CAM research. Challenges to the application of RCT methods to CAM can be categorised as either practical or methodological in nature. This chapter will address practical issues of interest before considering the methodological challenges facing the application of the RCT in CAM.

Practical issues in RCT CAM research

Practical issues facing RCT CAM research include inadequate research infrastructure, little incentive for practitioners to do research and poor funding, all of which inhibit both the development of research rigour and the retention of researchers in the field (Linde et al. 1997, Ernst 2001a, Nahin and Straus 2001, Ernst 2003, McCarthy 2002, Linde et al. 2001a, Spencer 1999). Some of these barriers are also problems for research in orthodox medicine (Stewart 2003, Gunn 2002).

Research is generally time-consuming and the often small effect sizes anticipated in CAM research may make trials larger and more expensive than those for conventional treatments (Linde and Jonas 1999). Even the preliminary research necessary prior to RCTs can be restrained by these factors. Basic laboratory-based research in CAM is essential, but costly. A good example is the development of techniques to standardise the amount of active ingredient(s) from plants. Even companies that have the expertise and finances to invest in developing the reproducible extraction techniques needed to ensure standard doses may find little incentive to invest their money for a patent. Seeking a patent may not secure exclusive market advantage given that natural products are widely available over the counter (Linde et al. 2001b, Eskinazi 1998).

Moreover, it is difficult for CAM producers to compete in the research field against large pharmaceutical companies providing products for the same indication (Linde and Jonas 1999). For example, in Australia atorvastatin and simvastatin, both lipid-lowering agents, were ranked first and second respectively in the top ten generic medications by value in 2003/4 (Australian Prescriber 2005). For each of these drugs there were approximately 7 million prescriptions subsidised by government expenditure of 397 million Australian dollars and 364 million Australian dollars respectively through the Pharmaceutical Benefits Scheme (Australian Prescriber 2005).[1] In contrast, in order to obtain the CAM alternative, policosanol, which has some evidence of efficacy (Varady et al. 2003), Australian patients must bear the full cost.

Unlike conventional medical research, complementary systems of care are not usually integrated with the national health system, so patients pay for consultations, investigations and treatments themselves. Therefore, funding for trials needs to include the cost of the therapy in addition to the legal and insurance issues that need to be considered when practitioners are not regulated (Mason et al. 2002).

These practical difficulties are only a selection of those facing CAM RCT research (for a more extensive discussion of such practical challenges facing the more general CAM research field see Cohen, Chapter 6). In the next section of this chapter, some core methodological issues facing those looking to develop CAM RCTs are discussed.

Methodological issues in RCT CAM research

Unlike the practical issues facing those interested in developing a rigorous evidence base for CAM using RCTs, methodological challenges are often unique to CAM research and require more consideration. Here I limit my discussion to identifying a number of methodological issues that I consider key to the further development of the field.

Paradigm clash

Orthodox medicine derives from a reductionist approach to the world and how it operates, that is, a belief that there is linear cause and effect of illness and that mechanisms of health and illness can be understood by breaking systems down into their smallest components for study. This is summarised by Patel as the 'Cartesian dichotomy between mind and body and a mono-etiological view of health and disease and its treatment' (1987).

In general, the holistic care of complementary systems involves different, usually multi-factorial, paradigms to orthodox medicine to explain causes of health and illness. CAM also embraces highly individualised approaches to diagnosis and treatment of patients, with an emphasis on boosting the body's own healing powers and viewing the patient as a whole being with physical, mental, social and spiritual needs (Coulter 2003). These therapies often have alternative conceptualisations of the human body that cannot be understood in biomedical terms (Adams and Tovey 2000), such as the existence of *qi* in traditional Chinese medicine (TCM) or *chakras* in Hindu philosophy.

This clash of world views is illustrated well by Patel's rhetorical questions: 'What, one wonders, would a [conventional medical] doctor do to treat a patient diagnosed as having an imbalance in the lesser Yin channel of the leg, a hardening of one of the 12 pulses taken at the wrist or a seasonal imbalance whose sound was "kung"?' (Patel 1987: 173). Similarly, a conventional researcher may perceive themselves are performing an RCT of traditional acupuncture or of spiritual healing, whereas practitioners and patients may view the same research as testing ancient theories of life forces or spiritual energies (Ernst 2003).

The RCT method can be seen as deriving from and therefore as favouring orthodox medicine and as inherently at odds with complementary holistic approaches to health care (Patel 1987, Lewith et al. 1996, Vickers 1998, Nahin and Straus 2001, Mason et al. 2002, Ernst 2003). Not surprisingly, there exists an inherent unease among some CAM practitioners/researchers regarding adoption of the reductionist RCT method to investigate CAM (Rothfield 1999, Thompson 2004). This unease is the nub of the paradigm clash between the two types of approaches to health, disease and healing. Given that RCTs are the best method to evaluate whether a treatment is effective, this clash is a problem that needs to be addressed and it underlies most of the other challenges explored in this chapter.

A vital starting point to address this problem is to involve researchers who are familiar with trial techniques as well as both orthodox and CAM therapies (Hoffer 2001). It may be that an individual possesses a range of appropriate skills and knowledge. For example, many conventional doctors also practise homoeopathy in the United Kingdom (Lewith et al. 2001) and acupuncture practice is widespread amongst the medical profession in Australia (Pirotta et al. 2002). Another approach is to utilise a range of experts from the outset of the study including those from the CAM therapy, orthodox medicine and others with expertise in designing and conducting RCTs. This will help ensure that the research questions and the trial design address issues relevant to each paradigm. Improper methodological restrictions placed on an intervention due to a lack of concern for its practical application may threaten the construct validity of the trial in the opinion of its practitioners (Caspi et al. 2004). Examples of this issue are discussed later in this chapter.

Trials may be designed to test integrated multifaceted whole complementary systems, rather than a single component of that system, otherwise 'researchers risk imposing a reductionist bias as to what constitutes a whole, evaluable treatment' (Levin et al. 1997: 1089). If a clearly defined and clinically relevant end point is applied (Nahin and Straus 2001, Smith 1995), trial protocols can be developed using CAM diagnosis and treatment, without developing a conventional understanding of the mechanism of action. These approaches are outlined in greater detail in the following sections.

Types of research questions asked

Formulating a clear research question is a vital initial step in conducting all good quality research. The question must be answerable, explicit, focused and practicable. An additional dimension in CAM research is whether the question posed is valid (Vickers et al. 1997). In this instance, validity may depend on one's point of reference. CAM practitioners may only view a research question that tests an entire CAM system as valid, wherein the diagnosis and treatment in all its possible complexity are true to the system being tested. On the other hand, conventional medical practitioners may be comfortable to adopt therapies from CAM systems, test individual components outside of their usual context and then incorporate those found to be effective into their own armamentarium. For example, a specific modality of a CAM system of healing may be applied to a Western diagnosis, such as using acupuncture to treat depression (Lewith et al. 1996, Vickers 1998, Nahin and Straus 2001). An even more reductionist approach would be to isolate one aspect of an alternative intervention, such as a specific herb, and apply it to a Western diagnosis (Nahin and Straus 2001). However, this approach does not validate or invalidate the whole complementary system.

There may be a lack of relevance of the trial question and therapy to clinical practice (Spencer 1999), particularly in homoeopathy, herbal medicine and acupuncture, where many trials do not represent the diagnoses and treatment combinations used in practice (Linde and Jonas 1999, Linde et al. 2001b, Linde et al. 2001c, Nahin and Straus 2001). Examples are when orthodox medicinal diagnostic criteria are applied to enrol participants for an RCT testing one particular acupuncture point (such as P6 for morning sickness [Vickers 1996]) or the orthodox diagnosis of hayfever and the testing of a standardised homoeopathic treatment (Reilly et al. 1986). A systematic review of trials using the single acupuncture point, P6, has found this to be effective therapy for nausea and vomiting (Vickers 1996). Yet, while this research question may be of interest to medical doctors, no acupuncturist would use this point in isolation. TCM practitioners, in addition to needling additional acupuncture points, may also draw on Chinese herbs, cupping, dietary changes, exercise (t'ai chi or qi gong) or moxibustion to treat the problem (Margolin et al. 1998, Linde and Jonas 1999, Nahin and Straus 2001). Designing a trial with a simplistic CAM intervention may reflect a desire to test the integration of complementary and orthodox medicines or a lack of understanding of the complex clinical underpinning of systems of complementary therapies. An unsuccessful trial using this type of design could not be seen to reflect on the complementary system as a whole, as the question does not reflect upon how the therapy is practised in the real world.

An example of how careful consultation with RCT method experts, conventional practitioners and CAM practitioners may ensure the development of research questions that are meaningful to all clinicians and their patients is a recent trial testing Chinese herbs for irritable bowel syndrome (IBS) (Bensoussan et al. 1998). The trial design was developed by Chinese herbalists and orthodox physicians. While trial inclusion criteria were based on conventional diagnostic criteria, all participants in the three study groups consulted a Chinese herbalist, with one group receiving individualised herbal formulations and the second group a standard formula designed by Chinese herbalists. The final group received placebo preparations (Bensoussan et al. 1998).

Ideally, the research protocol of CAM RCTs should be acceptable to both conventional and CAM practitioners. A further step to ensure this would be to screen potential participants using both orthodox and CAM diagnostic techniques (Spencer 1999), including adequate time for patient assessment, as complementary practitioners usually spend more time with each patient than conventional medical practitioners (Joyce 1994).

Researchers could focus on presentations, such as tiredness, rather than specific Western medical diagnoses (Mason et al. 2002). This was the approach adopted in a recent RCT of acupuncture to reduce driver fatigue which measured both physiological changes and participants' subjective evaluations of their fatigue after prolonged driving exercise at high speed (Li et al. 2004).

Types of interventions tested

Historically, RCTs have been employed to test pharmaceuticals, where dosages can be standardised and identical placebos manufactured. The RCT intervention can thus be well defined and other researchers and clinicians know exactly what treatment was trialled. However, it is far from simple to apply this methodology to a complex CAM intervention, such as treatment for a chronic illness, which may involve all of diet, acupuncture, herbs, exercise and massage. In addition to the plethora of strands constituting the whole treatment, complex CAM interventions need to be studied as tailored individualised packages to be meaningful to CAM practitioners and their patients (Patel 1987, Lewith et al. 1996, Vickers 1998). For example, in the cases of homoeopathy or acupuncture, the same diagnosis may receive different treatment depending on the individual's characteristics, and, unlike the manner in which conventional medicine is usually practised, a therapist's extensive case-taking is time-consuming. Both of these features are a challenge to fit into an RCT design. What often occurs is that a standardised homoeopathic solution or placebo is tested with patients meeting a conventional medical diagnosis, such as hayfever (Reilly et al. 1986). A homoeopath's individualised treatments and extensive case-taking may be an important part of the therapeutic effect, yet these are omitted from the trial just described. This may reduce the likelihood of detecting a difference in outcome between the two groups in an RCT.

This issue of testing complex and mixed interventions has been addressed in conventional medicine. One method used to overcome these issues, and avoid paradigm clash, is to incorporate whole systems into trial design, akin to a 'black box' of interventions, where the package of an intervention is trialled pragmatically as a whole without an attempt to break down the intervention into component parts. The 'black box' approach allows for complex, highly individualised treatment, such as that undertaken in trials of counselling techniques or for diverse community interventions, such as public-health approaches to reduce rates of smoking (Levin et al. 1997, Vickers 1998).

This approach may prove difficult for conventional clinicians to accept when the therapy being tested does not have an established mode of action, or at least one recognised by biomedical practitioners (Patel 1987, Linde and Jonas 1999). While an understanding of the mechanisms of action of particular therapies should be pursued in research, the lack of such understanding is not a barrier to testing a therapy via an RCT. It should be noted that a lack of understanding of how an intervention works also occurs for some orthodox medicine – for example, the mechanism of paracetamol is still not understood (Prescott 2000).[2]

The black-box approach also allays concern that the importance of the CAM therapist in healing may be ignored or underdeveloped (Mason et al. 2002). An example of this style of pragmatic RCT includes a UK trial, which randomised patients with chronic headache to either their usual GP care or to totally individualised acupuncture treatment over three months (Vickers et al. 2004). Similarly, an Australian RCT of manipulative therapy and/or non-steroidal anti-inflammatory drugs (NSAIDs) in addition to usual GP care for acute low back pain, allowed the treating physiotherapists flexibility to individualise treatments within an agreed treatment algorithm in order to allow replication and accurate description of the trial intervention (Hancock et al. 2005).

Alternatively, it may be possible and desirable to establish an agreed standard for an intervention by involving CAM practitioners in the planning of the research. In an RCT of acupuncture for the treatment of cocaine addiction, US researchers were able to utilise a protocol established by the National Acupuncture Detoxification Association (Margolin et al. 1998). If expert consensus or guidelines are not available, preliminary studies may be necessary prior to undertaking an RCT, to establish dose optimisation and length of time for treatments (Berman and Chesney 2005).

Herbal therapies also present difficulties in RCTs due to lack of accepted standards, including purity, dosage and delivery systems (Woolf et al. 1997, Lie 2002). Furthermore, plants may have a variety of complex bioactive ingredients, so evaluation is more complex than with a 'pure' drug trial (Linde and Jonas 1999), and different plant preparations have different compositions and properties (Linde and Jonas 1999, Linde et al. 2001b).

For example, three different species of echinacea are used medicinally; sometimes the roots are used, sometimes the stems and leaves and sometimes both. One well-designed RCT has studied the effect of unrefined echinacea for the common cold and has carefully described the echinacea constituents by percent age and weight of each capsule (Barrett et al. 2002). However, as the extraction method and even the season when harvested may produce different phytochemical compositions, the external generalisability of the results of any such trial is uncertain (Turner et al. 2002).

Also highlighting the difficulty with standardisation, some preparations of garlic have low levels of allicin which is thought to be essential for its antithrombolytic and hypolipidaemic effects. This may explain why some trials of garlic to lower elevated serum cholesterol levels and reduce atherosclerotic plaque formation have produced negative results while others have been positive (Lin et al. 2001). In addition to improving external generalisability of trial results (Farah et al. 2000, Lin et al. 2001), the importance of standardisation and characterisation of herbs to ensure purity, absence of harmful contaminants and accurate labelling is obviously also crucial to guaranteeing patient safety, and the issue requires further CAM industry attention.

The expertise and experience of the provider of an intervention may also limit external generalisability of the RCT's results. This issue is not unique to CAM, as it may also affect trials of other physical interventions, such as surgery, or highly individualised interventions, such as counselling. Faced with such a limitation, those designing trials can also stratify by individual practitioner to overcome problems with non-standardised treatments (Mason et al. 2002). Alternatively, the intervention can be delivered by a wide range of practitioners, to increase external generalisability. The most important issue here is that any positive results should be demonstrable with other practitioners (Joyce 1994).

Choice of comparator and double blinding

Some of the real conundrums facing the application of RCTs for CAM include the choice of comparator group, the role of non-specific and placebo effects in healing and the difficulty of double blinding (Schulz et al. 1995, Hensley and Gibson 1998, Linde and Jonas 1999, Margolin et al. 1998, Vickers 1998, Nahin and Straus 2001, Mason et al. 2002, Lie 2002, Ernst 2003). Consumers are turning to CAM practitioners partly in response to the relatively long consultation times of these providers and the more personalised service they offer (Joyce 1994). Non-specific and placebo effects may be a more important component in the healing process in complementary than in conventional consultations. It is widely known that people may respond well to placebo treatments (meaning 'I shall please') (Oh 1994), although research has failed to identify a consistent group of placebo responders (Kaptchuk 2002). Generally, non-specific effects in healing refer to the ability of the body to heal (enhanced by expectation), regression to the mean (people present when they have extreme symptoms and then they regress naturally to improved health), or even self-delusion (Jonas and Levin 1999). Kaptchuk describes non-specific effects as being 'present in any patient-practitioner relationship, including attention, communication of concern, intense monitoring, diagnostic procedures, labelling of complaint, and alterations produced in a patient's expectancy, anxiety and relationship to the illness' (Kaptchuk 2002: 817).

Having a comparison group is one hallmark of RCT design and allows researchers to differentiate between a placebo response (and possibly non-specific effects, depending on the RCT design) and the effect of the treatment being tested. While the RCT environment is highly controlled, the existence of a control group also allows for measurement of the progress of the condition over time without use of the intervention being tested.

The type of comparator used will be determined by the research question. If the research question focuses upon identifying whether one system of approach to a problem (for example, homoeopathy) is more effective than another (for example, the usual care of a family doctor), then the choice of comparator becomes clear. Comparing a homoeopathic consultation to a family doctor visit, both in their entirety, allows comparison of the CAM practitioners' role and the consultation – both integral to the therapeutic process (Cant and Calnan 1991). To reduce this 'package' to its component parts and then subject one aspect to an RCT is conceived by CAM proponents as fundamentally missing the point of the holistic paradigm (Verhoef et al. 2005). However, if the research question posed is whether a specific component is effective (for example, a homoeopathic solution), then that aspect of the treatment should be the only difference between the two groups, and a placebo homoeopathic solution would be the comparator. It should be acknowledged that this design may make it more difficult to prove any treatment effect, as both groups may be expected to improve in a clinically meaningful way from their baseline status, due to non-specific and placebo effects. Small effect sizes, requiring larger sample sizes and possibly more time to detect, can be an issue in all trials and can add considerably to the cost of research.

Prior to undertaking a trial, it is important that there exists genuine uncertainty about whether the experimental treatment is effective, this is termed 'clinical equipoise'. As stated previously, the choice of comparison group depends on the type of research question posed. In general, an active control, such as 'usual treatment', is utilised if the research question is to examine the risks and benefits of the trial intervention against a known therapy or where it would not be ethical to withhold a therapy of known value where this exists. For example, in a trial of acupuncture for chronic headache, both groups received their usual care from their GP, but the intervention group also had twelve treatments of acupuncture (Vickers et al. 2004).

An active control may also be necessary where blinding is not possible, such as in massage or spinal manipulation. For example, in one study performed in an intensive-care unit, participants were randomised either to massage, aromatherapy or rest (Dunn et al. 1995). Furthermore, a placebo control is used with regard to questions of efficacy, or in CAM research, to test whether the non-specific aspects of the treatment rather that the specific physiological aspects are responsible for any treatment effects detected (Caspi et al. 2004). For example, in an RCT of TCM for IBS, the presence of a third group, which also received an individual consultation with a TCM practitioner but only placebo medicine, allowed the researchers to control for any non-specific effects of the consultation (Bensoussan et al. 1998).

One challenge in conducting RCTs in some CAMs is the difficulty or impossibility of blinding either researchers/practitioners or their participants or both to the intervention group to which they are assigned. It can be appreciated that if blinding is not possible, then investigators' or patients' negative or positive views of the therapy may be a source of bias. Blinding is a particular issue, not only with acupuncture and physical therapies such as chiropractic, meditation, yoga and massage but also with some herbs that have a strong taste or an effect on skin or urine odour. Where blinding is not possible, researchers can use other types of comparators in pragmatic trials such as conventional medical practice as a control (usual care) (Vickers 1998, Mason et al. 2002).

Non-blinded trials require even more vigilance against bias than RCTs where blinding is possible. In circumstances where blinding of researchers and participants regarding their therapeutic group allocation is not possible, blinding of outcome assessors may still be available and is certainly recommended. Other checks for bias can be used in the design. In a chronic headache and acupuncture trial comparing usual GP care to usual GP care *and* acupuncture (Vickers et al. 2004) the treating GPs were at risk of performance bias, whereby they may have treated patients differently if they knew the group allocation. To deal with this, GPs were not informed of their patients' allocation to either the acupuncture group or the non-acupuncture group, and the patients were specifically asked not to discuss such details with their doctor. Also, patients could have been affected by response bias (they may have modified their response on outcomes assessments if they considered their doctor as potentially able to view their answers). In order to deal with this potential response bias; this particular RCT design employed the following three features: patients were expressly and repeatedly informed that their treating GP would not see their responses; all contact with the research team was via telephone to reduce social bias; and finally, the main question measuring the outcome was repeated at several time points (Vickers et al. 2004).

Researchers have been creative in their efforts to minimise bias through difficulty in choice of comparator and the issue of successful double-blinding. One RCT used thyme and peppermint to disguise the distinctive taste of echinacea in capsules and the success of blinding was established by asking participants at their completion whether they thought they had been assigned to the echinacea or placebo capsules (Barrett et al. 2002).

An adequate placebo for acupuncture therapy represents a unique challenge. Three mechanisms are believed to account for the effects of acupuncture: (1) 'specific' effects due to the stimulation of particular acupoints; (2) non-specific physiological effects due to piercing of the skin, which induces alterations in microcirculation, local immune function and neurally mediated analgesia; and (3) non-specific psychological effects (Caspi et al. 2004).

This complexity of therapeutic mechanisms presents a challenge to rigorous research design. Biomedical research requires that an adequate placebo comparator mimic all mechanisms apart from the specific effects. However, it may not be appropriate to divide the CAM therapeutic encounter, with its emphasis on holistic approach, into specific and non-specific aspects. For instance, research questioning TCM patients has identified that the experience of talking to and being listened to by a TCM practitioner is rated by participants as different to that experienced in a biomedical consultation. The researchers conclude that this is due to the talking/listening being linked to the underlying holistic theory of TCM and this aspect of the consultation is not seen as independent from any specific effects. It is also argued that the use of placebo designs for complex interventions may not detect the entire specific effect and may therefore lead to an underestimate of the total treatment effect and possible false-negative results (Paterson and Dieppe 2005).

Within TCM, there is no concept of placebo or inert acupuncture. While the needling of 'sham' points (points considered to have no therapeutic activity) is often used as a control in trials, there is debate as to whether these controls are actually therapeutically inactive and their use may lead to false-negative RCT results (Paterson and Dieppe 2005). Needling traditional and sham points can elicit similar physiological responses, which include endorphin release and reduced brain cortical activity in areas that deal with pain signals (Assefi et al. 2005). Other researchers have chosen to use acupuncture points for another indication as a control; for example, points for relaxation in an RCT of acupuncture for overactive bladder (Emmons and Otto 2005).

Another approach has been to test true acupuncture against superficial needling at non-acupuncture points. In one trial using this method, participants rated the credibility of true and sham acupuncture at the conclusion of the trial. This trial demonstrated statistically significant differences in the primary outcome in knee arthritis between the true and placebo acupuncture groups, although both of these groups had improved outcomes over the waiting-list control group (Witt et al. 2005). The use of superficial needling as a control group is also questionable as the Japanese school of acupuncture advocates superficial needling as being therapeutically beneficial (Nahin and Straus 2001). When designing trials with sham acupuncture, researchers often test the credibility of the control group 'acupuncture' with a credibility questionnaire at the conclusion of the study (Melchart et al. 2005, Witt et al. 2005). Researchers should also consider controlling for the non-specific psychological effects of acupuncture, in an ear acupuncture RCT for cocaine addiction, participants in the control group had to sit quietly for forty minutes per day to control for the rest component of the active acupuncture group (Margolin et al. 1998).

Other physical therapies also present difficulty with choice of comparator and double blinding. An RCT of reflexology for palliative-care patients utilised standard foot massage as the control and excluded patients who had previous experience of either foot massage or reflexology. This design further attempts to minimise bias by administering the therapy via three different therapists assigned at random over six weeks as well as through the use of a blinded assessor (Cornbleet and Ross 2001).

Outcome measures

In general, there is a lack of adequate and appropriate standardised outcome measures in some types of CAM (Lewith et al. 1996, Vickers 1998, Lie 2002, Mason et al. 2002). One criticism of applying the RCT method to CAM is that the outcome measures chosen may not be meaningful to the CAM practitioner and CAM system of therapy (Long 2002). However, using CAM-relevant outcomes may result in outcomes that may not be 'sensible' in biomedical terms (for example, Bach flower remedy of water violet formula to increase serenity, not serum violet [Levin et al. 1997]). CAM therapies often aim for long-term and subtle effects which may be hard to measure (Levin et al. 1997) and adequate length of follow-up in CAM RCTs is essential – for example, in chronic illness where responses may be slow (Mason et al. 2002).

A US NIH quantitative-methods working group summarised their recommendations in this way: a dependent variable can be expressed in either orthodox or CAM terms, as long as its validity can be verified by experts and 'reliability can be ascertained regardless of the unconventionality of the phenomenon being assessed provided the respective complementary medical system has an identifiable, systematic and consistent set of rules for assigning values to quantify attributes of the phenomenon' (Levin et al. 1997: 1089). This situation is analogous to an RCT of a drug with an unknown mechanism of action, such as paracetamol (Prescott 2000).

Researchers designing CAM RCTs need to liaise closely with experts in all relevant fields to ensure outcomes satisfy both CAM and orthodox practitioners. Trial designs could allow for a broad range of outcome measures to capture a wide range of symptoms such as personal growth or spiritual change (perhaps using qualitative methods) or changes in lifestyle that promote wellness as a means of satisfying both CAM and conventional researchers. Measures could also include the human experience as an outcome to maintain holistic intent (Smith 1995, Levin et al. 1997, Mason et al. 2002, Verhoef et al. 2005) (for a more detailed discussion of the combination of qualitative methods and RCT method, see Verhoef and Vanderheyden, Chapter 5). While cure is important, researchers can also consider healthy lifestyle, emotional well-being or more satisfying relationships as an outcome measure and some subjective outcomes, such as pain, are now accepted in orthodox medicine (Knipschild 1993, Vickers 1998). For example, an intensive-care study of aromatherapy, massage and rest employed physical measures, observations of behaviour and patient assessment of mood, anxiety and ability to cope as outcome measures (Dunn et al. 1995). Researchers may account for participants' expectations and beliefs in treatments at the outset of a trial as an independent variable, particularly if they cannot be blinded (Spencer 1999, Lie 2002, Mason et al. 2002), and trials can be designed to assess the therapeutic relationship as well as other non-specific effects (Mason et al. 2002, Kaptchuk 2002). It may be that new validated tools need to be purpose-designed, as shown with research to develop a tool to measure holistic practice, a key feature of CAM (Long et al. 2000).

Conclusions

The widespread community use of CAM has forced conventional medical clinicians and health policy-makers to consider the value of alternative approaches to health care. As this chapter has highlighted, many important issues face CAM researchers in the application of the gold-standard method, RCTs, to test the efficacy of CAM treatments.

A key issue facing the application of RCT methods with regard to CAM is the clash of the reductionist viewpoint (conceiving of a linear path between cause and effect and promoting the isolation of single elements of medical systems for study) and the CAM viewpoint (fundamentally holistic and vitalist in its approach).

Creative advances in RCT design allow whole systems to be evaluated using pragmatic approaches, without an understanding of the underlying mechanism of action of the interventions. Research also continues in the development of validated outcome measures, which are meaningful to CAM practitioners and their patients. Despite ongoing difficulties and challenges, there are reasons to remain optimistic that further progress can be made in the application of RCT method to the study of CAM. Ultimately, all health-care practitioners and their patients will be beneficiaries of this process.

Notes

1 The Australian governments' pharmaceutical benefits scheme (PBS) provides subsidised access to a wide range of medicines for all Australian citizens. (For further information see http://www.health.gov.au/internet/Publishing.nsf/Content/Pharmaceutical+Benefits+Scheme+(PBS)–1>.)
2 Paracetamol is known as acetaminophen in the USA.

References

Adams, J. and Tovey, P. (2000) 'Complementary medicine and primary care: towards a grassroots focus', in P. Tovey (ed.) *Contemporary Primary Care: The Challenges of Change*, Buckingham: Open University Press.

Allen, C., Glasziou, P. and Del Mar, C. (1999) 'Bed rest: a potentially harmful treatment needing more careful evaluation', *Lancet*, 354 (9186): 1229–33.

Angell, M. and Jerome, P. (1998) 'Alternative medicine: the risks of untested and unregulated remedies', *New England Journal of Medicine*, 339 (12): 839–41.

Anonymous (2000) 'Complementary medicine: time for critical engagement', *Lancet*, 356 (9247): 2023.

Assefi, N., Sherman, K., Jacobsen, C., Goldberg, J., Smith, W. and Buchwald, D. (2005) 'A randomised clinical trial of acupuncture compared with sham acupuncture in fibromyalgia', *Annals of Internal Medicine*, 143 (1): 10–19.

Australian Prescriber (2005) 'Top 10 Drugs', *Australian Prescriber*, 28 (2): 37.

Baldwin, E. (2003) 'Time for a fresh look at complementary medicine', *British Medical Journal*, 26 (7402): 1322.

Barnes, P., Powell-Griner, E., McFann, K. and Nahin, R. L. (2004) 'Complementary and alternative medicine use among adults: United States, 2002', *Advance Data*, 27 (343): 1–19.

Barrett, B., Brown, R., Locken, K., Maberry, R., Bobula, J. and D'Alessio, D. (2002) 'Treatment of the common cold with unrefined echinacea: a randomized, double-blind, placebo-controlled trial', *Annals of Internal Medicine*, 137 (12): 939–46.

Begbie, S., Kerestes, Z. and Bell, D. (1996) 'Patterns of alternative medicine use by cancer patients', *Medical Journal of Australia*, 165 (10): 540–6.

Bensoussan, A., Talley, N., Hing, M., Menzies, R., Guo, A. and Ngu, M. (1998) 'Treatment of irritable bowel syndrome with Chinese herbal medicine: a randomized controlled trial', *Journal of the American Medical Association*, 280 (18): 1585–9.

Berman, B., Singh, B., Lao, L., Singh, B., Ferentz, K. and Hartnoll, S. (1995) 'Physicians' attitudes toward complementary or alternative medicine: a regional survey', *Journal of the American Board of Family Practice*, 8 (5): 361–6.

Berman, J. and Chesney, M. (2005) 'Complementary and alternative medicine in 2006: optimising the dose of the intervention', *Medical Journal of Australia*, 183 (11/12): 574–5.

Cant, S. and Calnan, M. (1991) 'On the margins of the medical marketplace? An exploratory study of alternative practitioners' perceptions', *Sociology of Health and Illness*, 13 (1): 39–57.

Caspi, O., Stellhorn, C. and Connor, M. (2004) 'Sham in CAM: the anatomy and physiology of control and sham in complementary and alternative medicine research', *Evidence-Based Integrative Medicine*, 1 (4): 233–40.

Chen, H. and Ma, B. (2001) 'Research funds for complementary medicine', *Lancet*, 357 (9272): 1982.

Cohen, M., Penman, S., Pirotta, M. and Da Costa, C. (2005) 'The integration of complementary therapies in Australian general practice: results of a national survey', *Journal of Alternative and Complementary Medicine*, 11 (6): 995–1004.

Cornbleet, M. and Ross, C. (2001) 'Research in complementary medicine is essential', *British Medical Journal*, 322 (7288): 736–7.

Coulter, A. (2003) 'Killing the goose that laid the golden egg?', *British Medical Journal*, 326 (7402): 1280–1.

Dobson, R. (2003) 'Half of general practices offer patients complementary medicine', *British Medical Journal*, 327 (7426): 1250.

Doll, R. (1998) 'Controlled trials: the 1948 watershed', *British Medical Journal*, 317 (7167): 1217–20.

Dunn, C., Sleep, J. and Collett, D. (1995) 'Sensing an improvement: an experimental study to evaluate the use of aromatherapy, massage and periods of rest in an intensive care unit', *Journal of Advanced Nursing*, 21 (1): 34–40.

Emmons, S. L. and Otto, L. (2005) 'Acupuncture for overactive bladder: a randomized controlled trial', *Obstetrics and Gynecology*, 106 (1): 138–43.

Eisenberg, D., Kessler, R., Foster, C., Norlock, F., Calkins, D. and Delbanco, T. (1993) 'Unconventional medicine in the United States: prevalence, costs and patterns of use', *New England Journal of Medicine*, 328 (4): 246–52.

Ernst, E. (2000) 'Prevalence of use of complementary/alternative medicine: a systematic review', *Bulletin of the World Health Organisation*, 78 (2): 252–7.

—— (2001a) 'Complementary and alternative medicine', *Lancet*, 357 (9258): 802–3.

—— (2001b) 'Complementary therapies in palliative cancer care', *Cancer*, 91 (11): 2181–5.

—— (2003) 'Obstacles to research in complementary and alternative medicine', *Medical Journal of Australia*, 179 (6): 279.

Eskinazi, D. (1998) 'Factors that shape alternative medicine', *Journal of the American Medical Association*, 280 (18): 1621–3.

Farah, M., Edwards, R., Lindquist, M., Leon, C. and Shaw, D. (2000) 'International monitoring of adverse health effects associated with herbal medicines', *Pharmacoepidemiology and Drug Safety*, 9 (2): 105–12.

Finkelstein, A. and Rao, G. (2005) 'Levels of evidence: how they help in applying study findings to clinical practice [language of evidence: defining the terms of evidence-based medicine]', *The Journal of Family Practice*, 54 (12): 1032.

Fontanarosa, P. and Lundberg, G. (1998) 'Alternative medicine meets science', *Journal of the American Medical Association*, 280 (18): 1618–19.

Gardiner, P. and Wornham, W. (2000) 'Recent review of complementary and alternative medicine used by adolescents', *Current Opinion in Pediatrics*, 12 (4): 298–302.

Gunn, J. (2002) 'Should Australia develop primary care research networks?', *Medical Journal of Australia*, 177 (2): 63–6.

Hancock, M., Maher, C., Latimer, J., McLachlan, A., Cooper, C. and Day, R. (2005) 'Manipulative therapy and/or NSAIDs for acute low back pain: design of a randomised controlled trial', *BMC Musculoskeletal Disorders*, 6 (57).

Harris, P. and Rees, R. (2000) 'The prevalence of complementary and alternative medicine use among the general population: a systematic review of the literature', *Complementary Therapies in Medicine*, 8 (2): 88–96.

Hensley, M. and Gibson, P. (1998) 'Promoting evidence-based alternative medicine', *Medical Journal of Australia*, 169 (11–12): 573–4.

Hoffer, J. (2001) 'Proof versus plausibility: rules of engagement for the struggle to evaluate alternative cancer therapies', *Canadian Medical Association Journal*, 164 (3): 351–3.

Jacobs, B., Bent, S., Tice, J., Blackwell, T. and Cummings, S. (2005) 'An internet-based randomized, placebo-controlled trial of kava and valerian for anxiety and insomnia', *Medicine*, 84 (4): 197–207.

Jonas, W. and Levin, J. (eds) (1999) *Essentials of Complementary and Alternative Medicine*, Baltimore, Md.: Lippincott, Williams and Wilkins.

Joyce C. (1994) 'Placebo and complementary medicine', *Lancet*, 344 (8932): 1279–81.

Kaptchuk, T. (2002) 'The placebo effect in alternative medicine: can the performance of a healing ritual have clinical significance?', *Annals of Internal Medicine*, 136 (11): 817–25.

Kerr, D. (1996) 'In search of truth', *Journal of the Royal College of Physicians*, 30 (5): 405.

Knipschild, P. (1993) 'Alternative thoughts on the methodology of clinical trials', *British Medical Journal*, 306 (6894): 1706–7.

Levin, J., Glass, T., Kushi, L., Schuk, J., Steele, L. and Jonas, W. (1997) 'Quantitative methods in research on complementary and alternative medicine: a methodology manifesto', *Medical Care*, 35 (11): 1079–94.

Lewith, G. T., Kenyon, J. and Lewis, P. (1996) *Complementary Medicine: An Integrated Approach*, Oxford: Oxford University Press.

Lewith, G. T., Hyland, M. and Gray, S. F. (2001) 'Attitudes to and use of complementary medicine among physicians in the United Kingdom', *Complementary Therapies in Medicine*, 9 (3): 167–72.

Li, Z., Jiao, K., Chen, M. and Wang, C. (2004) 'Reducing the effects of driving fatigue with magnitopuncture stimulation', *Accident Analysis and Prevention*, 36 (4): 501–5.

Lie, D. (2002) 'Second international scientific conference on complementary, alternative and integrative medicine research', *Medscape Primary Care*, 4 (1).

Lin, M., Nahin, R., Gershwin, M., Longhurst, J. and Wu, K. (2001) 'State of complementary and alternative medicine in cardiovascular, lung, and blood research: executive summary of a workshop', *Circulation*, 103 (16): 2038–41.

Linde, K. and Jonas, W. (1999) 'Evaluating complementary and alternative medicine: the balance of rigor and relevance', in W. Jonas and J. Levin (eds) *Essentials of Complementary and Alternative Medicine*, Baltimore, Md.: Lippincott, Williams and Wilkins, pp. 51–71.

Linde, K., Clausius, N., Ramirez, G., Melchart, D., Eitel, F. and Hedges, L. (1997) 'Are the clinical effects of homoeopathy placebo effects? A meta-analysis of placebo-controlled trials', *Lancet*, 350 (9503): 834–43.

Linde, K., Vickers, A., Hondras, M., ter Riet, G., Thormaehlen, T. and Berman, B. (2001a) 'Systematic reviews of complementary therapies – an annotated biography. Part 1: acupuncture', *BMC Complementary and Alternative Medicine*, 1 (3).

Linde, K., ter Riet, G., Hondras, M., Vickers, A., Saller, R. and Melchart, D. (2001b) 'Systematic reviews of complementary therapies – an annotated biography. Part 2: Herbal medicine', *BMC Complementary and Alternative Medicine*, 1 (5).

Linde, K., Hondras, M., Vickers, A., ter Riet, G. and Melchart, D. (2001c) 'Systematic reviews of complementary therapies – an annotated biography. Part 3: Homoeopathy', *BMC Complementary and Alternative Medicine*, 1 (4).

Long, A. (2002) 'Outcome measurement in complementary and alternative medicine: unpicking the effects', *Journal of Alternative and Complementary Medicine*, 8 (6): 777–86.

Long, A., Mercer, G. and Hughes, K. (2000) 'Developing a tool to measure holistic practice: a missing dimension in outcomes measurement within complementary therapies', *Complementary Therapies in Medicine*, 8 (1): 26–31.

McCarthy, M. (2002) 'US panel calls for more support of alternative medicine', *Lancet*, 359 (9313): 1213.

MacLennan, A. H., Wilson, D. and Taylor, A. (2002) 'The escalating cost and prevalence of alternative medicine', *Preventive Medicine*, 35 (2): 166–73.

Margolin, A., Avants, S. and Kleber, H. (1998) 'Investigating alternative medicine therapies in randomized controlled trials', *Journal of American Medical Association*, 280 (18): 1626–8.

Mason, S., Tovey, P. and Long, A. (2002) 'Evaluating complementary medicine: methodological challenges of randomised controlled trials', *British Medical Journal*, 325: 832–4.

Melchart, D., Streng, A., Hoppe, A., Brinkhaus, B., Witt, C. and Wagenpfeil, S. (2005) 'Acupuncture in patients with tension-type headache: randomised controlled trial', *British Medical Journal*, 331 (7513): 376–82.

Nahin, R. and Straus, S. (2001) 'Research into complementary and alternative medicine: problems and potential', *British Medical Journal*, 322 (7279): 161–4.

Oh, V. (1994) 'The placebo effect: can we use it better?', *British Medical Journal*, 309 (6947): 69–70.

Patel, M. (1987) 'Evaluation of holistic medicine', *Social Science and Medicine*, 24 (2): 169–75.

Paterson, C. and Dieppe, P. (2005) 'Characteristic and incidental (placebo) effects in complex interventions such as acupuncture', *British Medical Journal*, 330 (7501): 1202–5.

Pirotta, M., Farish, S., Kotsirilos, V. and Cohen, M. (2002) 'Characteristics of Victorian general practitioners who practise complementary therapies', *Australian Family Physician*, 31 (12): 1133–8.

Pirotta, M., Gunn, J., Chondros, P., Grover, S., O'Malley, P. and Hurley, S. (2004) 'Effect of lactobacillus in preventing post-antibiotic vulvovaginal candidiasis: a randomised controlled trial', *British Medical Journal*, 329 (7465): 548–52.

Porter, R. (1997) *The Greatest Benefit to Mankind: A Medical History of Humanity from Antiquity to the Present*, London: HarperCollins.

Prescott, L. (2000) 'Paracetamol: past, present, and future', *American Journal of Therapeutics*, 7 (2): 143–7.

Reilly, D., Taylor, M., McSharry, C. and Aitchison, T. (1986) 'Is homoeopathy a placebo response? Controlled trial of homoeopathic potency, with pollen in hayfever as a model', *Lancet*, 2 (8512): 881–5.

Rothfield, P. (1999) 'How important is the placebo effect: the scientific evaluation of complementary medicines', *Diversity*, 1 (17): 14–16.

Schulz, K., Chalmers, I., Hayes, R. and Altman, D. (1995) 'Empirical evidence of bias: dimensions of methodological quality associated with estimates of treatment effects in controlled trials', *Journal of the American Medical Association*, 273 (5): 408–12.

Smith, I. (1995) 'Commissioning complementary medicine', *British Medical Journal*, 310 (6988): 1151–2.

Spencer, J. (1999) 'Essential issues in complementary/alternative medicine', in J. Spencer and J. Jacobs (eds) *Complementary/Alternative Medicine: An Evidence-Based Approach*, St Louis, Miss.: Mosby.

Stewart, P. M. (2003) 'Improving clinical research', *British Medical Journal*, 327 (7422): 999–1000.

Thomas, K., Coleman, P. and Nicholl, J. (2003) 'Trends in access to complementary or alternative medicines via primary care in England: 1995–2001. Results from a follow-up national survey', *Family Practice*, 20 (5): 575–7.

Thompson, T. (2004) 'Can the caged bird sing? Reflections on the application of qualitative research methods to case study design in homeopathic medicine', *BMC Medical Research Methodology*, 4 (4).

Turner, R. (2002) 'Echinacea for the common cold: can alternative medicine be evidence-based medicine?', *Annals of Internal Medicine*, 137 (12): 1001–2.

Varady, K., Wang, Y. and Jones, P. (2003) 'Role of policosanols in the prevention and treatment of cardiovascular disease', *Nutrition Reviews*, 61 (11): 376–83.

Verhoef, M., Lewith, G., Ritenbaugh, C., Boon, H., Fleishman, S. and Leis, A. (2005) 'Complementary and alternative medicine whole systems research: beyond identification of inadequacies of the RCT', *Complementary Therapies in Medicine*, 13 (3): 206–12.

Vickers, A. (1996) 'Can acupuncture have specific effects on health? A systematic review of acupuncture antiemesis trials', *Journal of the Royal Society of Medicine*, 89 (6): 303–11.

—— (1998) *Examining Complementary Medicine*, London: Stanley Thornes.

Vickers, A., Cassileth, B., Ernst, E., Fisher, P., Goldman, P. and Jonas, W. (1997) 'How should we research unconventional therapies?', *International Journal of Technology Assessment in Health Care*, 13 (1): 111–21.

Vickers, A., Rees, R., Zollman, C., McCarney, R., Smith, C. and Ellis, N. (2004) 'Acupuncture of chronic headache disorders in primary care: randomised controlled trial and economic analysis', *Health Technology Assessment*, 8 (48): 1–35.

White, A., Resch, K. and Ernst, E. (1997) 'Complementary medicine: use and attitudes among general practitioners', *Family Practice*, 14 (4): 302–6.

Witt, C., Brinkhaus, B., Jena, S., Linde, K., Streng, A. and Wagenpfeil, S. (2005) 'Acupuncture in patients with osteoarthritis of the knee: a randomised trial', *Lancet*, 366 (9480): 136–43.

Woolf, S., Bell, H., Berman, B., Brenner, Z., Hoffman, F. and Hudgings, C. (1997) 'Clinical practice guidelines in complementary and alternative medicine', *Archives of Family Medicine*, 6 (2): 149–54.

Chapter 5

Combining qualitative methods and RCTs in CAM intervention research

Marja J. Verhoef and Laura C. Vanderheyden

Introduction

The RCT is a strong research design to address questions of intervention effectiveness and one which is key to establishing an evidence base for CAM. RCTs have some limitations, however, when applied to some CAM interventions.[1] RCTs only address the question of whether an intervention works and not the process by which an intervention works or the context in which it works best. In many CAM interventions, process and context are fundamental to effective treatment and positive outcomes. Process describes how an intervention is delivered and how a patient actively participates in healing while on a personal transformative journey. Context describes the healing environment, the role of patient and practitioner expectations and the meaning of an intervention to a patient (Verhoef et al. 2002). Acknowledging these components in CAM-intervention research will provide insight into how and why CAM healing systems can provide a range of physical, emotional and spiritual treatment benefits to many patients.

In this chapter we examine how qualitative research can complement the RCT design to advance understanding of how, when and why CAM works. The purpose of qualitative research is to explore patient experiences, behaviours and beliefs in depth and to advance comprehensive theories that are grounded in patient-centred data. Complementing RCTs with qualitative research can address the limitations of the RCT design when applied to CAM interventions by capturing the essential components of process and context. We describe how qualitative and quantitative (RCT) designs differ and why we feel that these two seemingly different research approaches may be combined to increase the validity of CAM intervention research. We also present reasons for combining RCTs with qualitative research and outline a range of strategies for combining the two research approaches. Finally, through the use of examples, we discuss the many advantages this combined approach can bring and consider some of the barriers and challenges to combining qualitative research approaches with RCTs.

Combining research methods: degrees of methodological integration

Before exploring these issues in more detail, it is first necessary to address the varied terminology that exists in the literature regarding combining qualitative and quantitative research methods. Many different labels have been employed to describe research approaches that use both qualitative and quantitative methods, depending on the level of methodological integration. Labels include: mixed methods (Tashakkori and Teddlie 2003); combined methods (Buchanan 1992); integrated methods (Coyle and Williams 2000); methodological pluralism (Barker and Pistrang 2005); and multi-method research (Stange 2004). For the purposes of this chapter we would like to delineate between degrees of methodological integration in such research. We reserve the term 'multi-method' for less integrated designs, for example when a qualitative component is simply added to an RCT but the data collection, analysis and interpretation are kept relatively separate. For more integrated designs where qualitative and quantitative methods inform each other at many and sometimes all phases of the research (depending on the purpose/question) we use the term 'combined methods'. It is important to keep in mind that there is a wide range of potential ways in which the two research approaches can be combined and various ways in which methodological integration can and has been classified.

Differences between qualitative and quantitative research

Quantitative research, in particular RCTs, is well suited to answering questions such as whether an intervention works for a well-defined group of individuals or how one intervention compares to another intervention. Meanwhile, qualitative research is well suited to describing and exploring patient experiences, the meanings an intervention has for a patient and the process by which a patient heals (for detailed discussion see Aldridge, Chapter 1). Quantitative research methods are often aligned with a (post-) positivist epistemology and an objectivist ontology: reality is fixed and singular and can only be found through objective observation. The researcher is separate from the researched, collects objective data through the use of standardised, valid and reliable instruments and reduces and analyses numerical data through the use of statistical tests. Qualitative research methods are often aligned with an interpretivist epistemology and a constructionist ontology: reality is subjective and multiple and meaning is created through social interaction and is therefore constantly being revised. Following this paradigm, the researcher is a core tool in the research process and actively engages with those being researched to create data grounded in context. Textual data are reduced through coding, categorising and comparison. The differences between the two approaches are summarised in Table 5.1.

Examining Table 5.1, it would appear that such different methods cannot be combined and, in fact, the recent trend to combine qualitative and quantitative research methods is not without controversy. One line of reasoning promotes what can be termed the incompatibility thesis: qualitative and quantitative research methods are based on fundamentally opposing philosophical assumptions regarding epistemology (view of knowing and the relationship between knower and to-be-known) and ontology (view of reality) and therefore cannot be combined. In contrast, there is also the argument that qualitative and quantitative methods and paradigms are different and

Table 5.1 Description of qualitative and quantitative research approaches

Research approach	Qualitative	Quantitative
Ontology (nature of reality)	Constructionist	Objectivist
Epistemology (theory of knowledge)	Interpretivist	Positivist
Research purpose	To understand complex phenomena; to generate new ideas; to have personal, social, institutional and/or organizational impact (Newman et al. 2003)	To predict, measure change; to add to knowledge base (generalize); to test ideas (Newman et al. 2003)
Research question	What? Why? (classification/ meaning)	How many? Strength of association (enumeration/ causation)
Design	Flexible: natural setting, process oriented	Scientific rigor: highly controlled (outcome oriented), often experimental
Reasoning	Inductive	Deductive
Hypotheses	Generation	Testing
Sampling	Purposive (evolving)	Statistical (predetermined)
Data collection	In-depth interviews, focus groups, observation	Structured interviews, questionnaires, administrative records
Measurement	Researcher as instrument ('insider view'/subjective)	Psychosocial/physiological instruments ('outsider view'/objective
Data reduction	Words/categories/themes	Numerical, imposed codes
Data analysis	Coding/categorizing/ comparing	Statistical inference/ statistical estimation

logically independent (Patton 1990, Sandelowski 2000) and, therefore, there is no issue with combining these methods.

Somewhere in the middle of this continuum of controversy lies the pragmatist's argument, which looks to the strengths of both methods to overcome the weaknesses in each and gives primacy to the research question to dictate which methods may be most appropriate in a given situation. Bryman (2001) indicates that positivism/objectivism is only a tendency of quantitative research and interpretivism/constructivism is only a tendency of qualitative research – the assumptions are not definitive. This school of thought acknowledges there are undoubtedly differences between qualitative and quantitative research approaches but such differences, it is suggested, should not be exaggerated to the point where the methods may not be combined or used to complement one another. In line with this stance, we argue that the research purpose, the research question and the need for internal, external and model validity should be the deciding factors regarding which research methods should be used to approach a research problem.

Combining research methods and CAM

In addition to, and sometimes instead of, CAM, the notion of integrative medicine has become increasingly popular (Kligler and Lee 2004), reflecting the fact that many people use both conventional and CAM treatments either in a combined or an integrated fashion (Adams et al. 2003; Barnes et al. 2004). Integrative (or holistic) medicine has been defined as 'a balanced, whole person approach that involves a synthesis of conventional medicine, CAM modalities and/or other traditional medical systems, with the aim of prevention and healing as a basic foundation' (Kligler and Lee 2004). In this context, it is abundantly clear that if we wish to evaluate CAM (and integrative medicine), an integrated assessment approach is needed that consists of quantitative and qualitative approaches.

It is of great importance that investigative methods to assess CAM are valid. Previously, one of the current authors and her co-investigators have described the need for internal, external and model validity in CAM intervention research (Verhoef et al. 2005). Specifically, internal validity refers to the extent to which research results are free from systematic error. External validity describes the ability to generalise research results to a different context, and model validity concerns the extent to which the research approach respects the unique healing philosophy and therapeutic context of the intervention under investigation (Lewith et al. 2002). Model validity is of particular importance in CAM research, as many traditional research methods (for example, the RCT) were developed for biomedical interventions and, thus, are often inappropriate if applied directly to CAM interventions. If an RCT alone is used to evaluate a CAM intervention, the investigative approach does not have model validity, as among other reasons,[2] it does not allow the process and context of healing to be assessed.

It is clear that neither qualitative nor quantitative research methods *alone* can simultaneously achieve internal, external and model validity. While RCTs are often strong in terms of internal validity (the precision and control over extraneous variables), it is also the case that these same extraneous variables are essential to healing and, as such, controlling them will lessen the applicability of research results in the real world (external validity). Qualitative research is a strong approach for exploring patient experiences of an intervention and can achieve high model validity. Nevertheless, small sample sizes and context-bound results cannot provide adequate confirmatory evidence of effectiveness and are not necessarily appropriate to test hypotheses. When combined, qualitative research and the RCT can provide a flexible research design that can adequately capture whether an intervention works, how and in what context, in a manner that respects the unique healing philosophy of an intervention and that also produces generalisable results.

Reasons for combining qualitative research and the RCT

Qualitative and quantitative methods should not be combined under the assumption that 'more is better' (Sandelowski 2000) or that qualitative research is incomplete without quantitative research (Morse 1996). The need to combine methods arises not only from the requirement for high internal, external and model validity but also the demands of the specific research question. Four commonly identified reasons for combining methods, as they relate to the research question (Greene et al. 1989, Sandelowski 2000) have been outlined. These are briefly discussed below.

Convergence or confirmation

Seeking convergence, corroboration or correspondence of results from different methods to achieve convergent validation of the results is often mentioned as the most important reason for combining methods. Due to scarce resources, however, it has been a rare motivation in more recent research. This line of reasoning has also been labelled triangulation, but due to the many meanings this term carries, it is less useful (Morgan 1998).

Complementarity

Here, a combined-methods approach is employed with the aim of seeking elaboration, enhancement, illustration or clarification of the results from one method with the results from another method. Combining for this reason increases the interpretability, meaningfulness and validity of findings by capitalising on strengths inherent in one method and counteracting limitations or biases inherent in the other method (Sandelowski 2000). When assessing the effectiveness of CAM interventions, this is the most common reason for combining RCTs and qualitative research approaches. In CAM research, RCTs allow the potential for effective healing to be revealed while qualitative methods allow exploration of the process by which healing occurs, the context in which healing is optimised and the specific personal benefits of the intervention.

Development

Another objective for combining methods is to use the results from one method to help develop or inform the other method, where development is broadly construed to include sampling, implementation and measurement decisions. Development is a particularly relevant reason to combine when healing systems that include a variety of components (such as naturopathic medicine, or TCM) are being evaluated and when the research process requires several phases of exploration and testing.

Initiation

Finally, seeking the discovery of paradox and contradiction, new perspectives or frameworks and recasting of questions or results from one method with questions or results from the other method is a justified reason for a combined-method approach. Qualitative research and the RCT are based on distinct philosophical assumptions, but neither is seen as incorrect; they are just different. Combining both approaches in one study can initiate insights into how and why CAM works that would not be attainable without combining (Polit and Hungler 1999). Again, as for the justification of development, combining methods with the aim of initiation is extremely useful in the evaluation of healing systems with many varied components.

Greene et al. (1989) highlight that the array of reasons for combining qualitative and quantitative methods ranges from very restricted (convergence) to wide and flexible (initiation). In CAM intervention research, the latter reasons are becoming more and more important, due to the complexity of many healing systems. Accompanying these reasons for combining research methods are a number of strategies for accomplishing such combination at the grass-roots level. It is to these strategies that we now turn our attention.

Combined method design strategies

Basic forms of combination

Morgan (1998) describes four general forms of combining qualitative and quantitative research that are commonly accepted. These four forms are based on two principles, *priority* and *sequence*. Priority refers to the decision regarding whether a qualitative or a quantitative component will be the principal method for data collection, and sequence refers to the decision regarding the order of the qualitative and quantitative components. Taken together, there are four forms – dependent on which method is dominant and which is complementary and whether the complementary method precedes or follows the dominant method.

This typology is useful as it highlights important decisions that must be made when designing combined-methods research. Nevertheless, it ignores more integrated designs where the priority given to each approach is equal and qualitative and quantitative data collection and analysis occur simultaneously and inform each other at various stages (Creswell 2003). The typology is also too simple for complex CAM interventions that require a more complex design strategy – one that is more iterative and involves ongoing 'waves' of qualitative and quantitative research (Sandelowski 2000). For example, a study to assess the benefits of TCM for asthma could start with qualitative pilot work with past users to identify relevant outcomes. This pilot work could be followed by an RCT that employs those outcomes, which in turn could be followed by qualitative interviews with participants who did and did not respond well to explore the question of for which participants the treatment may be most beneficial and why. In such a design, qualitative research and the RCT are given equal priority and the design is more iterative than sequential.

Towards a whole system approach

Many CAM interventions are complex and consist of many varied components. For example, TCM comprises multiple components, such as acupuncture, herbal products and massage. However, acupuncture or massage therapy alone may also be considered to comprise multiple components, including the intervention, the patient–provider relationship, the context of healing and patient and practitioner expectations. In order to fully understand a CAM intervention, research must address the separate components, while allowing the system to remain intact (that is, not be reduced to its 'component' or 'active' parts). Due to synergy between the different components, it is apparent that the overall healing effect of CAM interventions can be greater than the sum of the healing effect of each component part.

CAM intervention research must therefore involve a continuous interplay between a variety of research methods, recognising that the creation of knowledge is a continuous and evolutionary process. Qualitative research should be combined with the RCT and other quantitative designs, both within and between individual projects and both methods should *always* be given equal priority.

CAM whole systems research is an emerging research framework specific for the investigation of the effectiveness of whole systems of health care, or interventions with many varied components (Verhoef et al. 2005). The aim is to employ appropriate research designs and methods so that all aspects of an internally consistent approach to treatment, or a whole system, can be assessed within its unique explanatory model (Ritenbaugh et al. 2003). Whole systems research must acknowledge an individualised, patient-centred and participatory approach to diagnosis and treatment as well as a process of healing that collaboratively combines patient and practitioner knowledge and skills, thus enhancing healing. Whole systems research follows a non-hierarchical, cyclical, flexible and adaptable process of inquiry, recognising that a combination of methods is required and that no one method (be it qualitative or quantitative) alone can adequately capture the meaning, process and outcomes of whole system interventions.

The multivariate conceptualisation of whole systems, including the patient–practitioner relationship, the context of healing, the individualised nature of diagnosis and treatment, patient and practitioner expectations and patient-centred outcomes, sets whole systems research apart from conventional biomedical research and the RCT. In this context, RCTs should ideally be adaptations of the classic RCT. For example, *pragmatic RCTs* allow for the assessment of individualised treatment approaches while maintaining control through randomisation. Contrastingly, *factorial RCTs* compare single modalities (for example, acupuncture) to a combination of modalities (for example, TCM) to allow for the assessment of multiple interaction effects between different treatment 'components'. Meanwhile, *preference RCTs* allow patients with strong treatment expectations or preferences to receive their preferred treatment, and patients with no treatment preference are randomised following usual procedures.

Combining qualitative research with an adapted RCT design can take several forms in whole systems research. Methods can be combined in an *iterative* fashion where the results of one approach continuously inform the development of another approach and vice versa. Or, qualitative methods can be nested in a dominant RCT to explore one specific component of the system. Generally, whole systems research is *holistic* as it is achieved by simultaneous integration of methods throughout the evaluation, building towards one integrated explanation of results. It might even be possible that such designs become *transformative* if primacy is given to value-based and action-oriented dimensions of this different research approach.

Examples of combined methods research for CAM

Over the past four years, several studies have been reported in which qualitative methods are combined with RCTs (Alraek and Baerheim 2001, Alraek and Baerheim 2003, Cohen-Katz et al. 2005, Mehling et al. 2005, Brazier et al. 2006). Below we briefly discuss these studies, highlighting their core features and focus. Referring back to the reasons for combined-methods research previously outlined, we can see that most of the following examples aim at complementing data collected in RCTs with qualitative methods. Some of the studies have elements of development, most have overlapping intentions. No examples of whole systems research have yet been published, but based on the increased attention to whole systems research and the workshops that have been offered in this area, it is likely that several studies are currently in progress.

Example 1: the art of living with HIV

In 2000, one of the current authors and her colleagues conducted an evaluation of a mind–body programme entitled 'The Art of Living with HIV' (Brazier et al. 2006) employing combined methods. The objective of this research was to assess the effectiveness of a two-week residential yogic breathing, movement and meditation programme aimed at improving mental health, health status and reducing stress among people living with HIV/AIDS. The residential programme was followed by once per week follow-up sessions (twelve weeks). The study design was a small RCT complemented by in-depth qualitative interviews to assess the perceived benefits of the programme. The RCT alone could not have addressed the research question, as the research team did not know in advance the range of relevant outcomes or the process that would be involved in participants' healing journey. The design was sequential, with equal priority given to each research approach.

Forty-seven participants completed the study and fourteen participants were interviewed after returning from the residential programme. Outcome measures included the mental health index (MHI), the MOS-HIV Health Survey, the daily stress inventory (DSI) and a fifty-eight-item checklist of common stressful events where respondents were asked to identify stressful events and the personal impact of each event that occurred. The results showed significant improvements as measured with the MHI and MOS-HIV one week after completion of the programme, but these differences were not sustained at six and twelve weeks. The DSI showed that participants in the treatment group identified significantly more stressors and a higher stress level than the control group at each time. By these results, the programme was a failure.

The qualitative results, however, showed that participants experienced a personal growth process following the intervention. 'Living' began to feel more meaningful and conscious. Participants were learning to feel everything, pleasant and unpleasant, with greater intensity – but this greater self-awareness also included greater awareness of changes, stress, pain and discomfort. Accepting and embracing these changes was not always comfortable and at times proved stressful.

When combined, the qualitative results were able to clarify the results of the RCT, which increased the validity of the study findings. Combining allowed the development of a more sensitive approach to preparing future participants for the programme and for more specific follow-up.

Example 2: holistic outcomes of TCM acupuncture for women with recurrent cystitis

Alraek and Baerheim (2001) sequentially collected qualitative data using an open-ended free-text questionnaire following an RCT to evaluate the effect of TCM acupuncture treatment in women with recurrent cystitis (Alraek and Baerheim 2003). The purpose of the qualitative questionnaire was to complement RCT results and to explore changes in health as reported by women in the treatment group.

Outcomes other than physiologic trial outcomes were identified, including normalised urination with better pressure during voiding and more complete bladder emptying, normalised bowel movements and less abdominal discomfort. In addition, many women reported more energy, reduced stress, better sleep and improvements in painful disorders. The illustrative descriptions provided by the women covered many areas of the body and described health changes that occurred in addition to curing the problem they came for, consistent with the ancient view of TCM as restoring harmony in the individual. The combining of qualitative research and the RCT provided a rigorous design that enhanced understanding of the intervention.

Example 3: mindfulness-based stress reduction for nurse stress and burnout

Cohen-Katz et al. (2005) iteratively collected quantitative and qualitative data in their pre-test and post-test waiting-list control-group design with randomisation to examine the impact of an eight-week mindfulness-based stress-reduction (MBSR) programme on nurse stress and burnout. Qualitative sources consisted of weekly evaluation forms, final evaluation forms, e-mails, interviews and a focus group. The stated reasons for qualitative data collection included: the small size of the treatment group (n=25), thus the need for other types of data; the need to explore the impact of MBSR in a more open-ended way; and the need to understand aspects of the intervention, such as self-care, self-awareness and therapeutic presence, which are difficult to capture with quantitative data.

In the process of data collection, new and unexpected qualitative data emerged, related in particular to the unsolicited emails the investigators received during and after the programme. Key themes of the qualitative analysis of these emails included reasons for participating in the programme, expected benefits, expected impact of MBSR on relationships and how to maintain the practice over time. Recognising the cyclical and evolutionary process of knowledge creation, the investigators appropriately identified several questions for future research – for example, the impact on family relationships and the work environment. Combining methods in this study therefore served multiple purposes: convergence of results from both approaches; elaborating on and clarifying results from both approaches (complementarity); and initiation of new ways of understanding how an MBSR programme may work through increasing the depth and breadth of inquiry.

Example 4: breathing therapy for chronic low back pain

Mehling et al. (2005) conducted a six to eight week (twelve sessions) RCT to assess the effect of breath therapy as compared to physical therapy on patients with chronic low back pain. During the intervention, all study participants kept a diary and received instructions:

> What was important for you today? Please feel free to share in your own words any commentaries about your treatment experience. . . . We would like to know your thoughts and feelings related to your therapy and therapist, whether you think any differently about your body, your back, your pain or life in general.
>
> (Mehling et al. 2005: 46)

Diary entries resulted in five main themes: functioning in daily life activities; exercise-related experiences; effect on emotions; insights about pain and coping; and relation to body and self. Major differences between the groups emerged with respect to effect on emotions and insights about pain and coping, with virtually no entries by control-group participants. The dominant RCT design provided a rigorous means to compare two treatment groups, while complementary qualitative data collection allowed participants to express in their own words how they benefited (or not) from the intervention and provided an opportunity to expand understanding of the impact of the intervention.

In all of the above examples, results emerged that would have remained hidden if qualitative methods and the RCT were not combined. Qualitative data collection added to an understanding of the process and context in which interventions were or were not effective and the meaning attached to the intervention, and in several studies new insights led to new research questions for future studies. In the first example, combining methods enhances our insight into the healing and treatment process. In all examples, combining methods allows the identification of outcomes that are relevant to the participants and not just the researchers.

An additional effect of combining qualitative research with the RCT, not mentioned above, is a context effect that is consistent with our observations that qualitative research itself may have a beneficial effect. Several participants in our qualitative research have commented on the therapeutic value of participating in qualitative data collection. Participants have mentioned that they appreciate the attention paid to them and the opportunity to be listened to, the importance placed on their individual experiences and the self-awareness that is created by talking through their feelings and reasons for those feelings (Verhoef 2005). However, while a benefit, this non-specific effect can also serve as a confounder of trial results when included in combined methods research, as the qualitative research may, in fact, change the intervention, which demonstrates the complexities of such research.

Barriers and challenges to combined methods research

Although there is great potential for combining qualitative research methods with a rigorous RCT design, the task is not easy and there remain many challenges. Combining methods can be very costly: varied data must be collected and analysed, which is unquestionably time-consuming and expensive. Specialised computer software programs may be needed to assist in both types of analysis. Further, combining methods not only requires expertise in both quantitative and qualitative research methods but also in combined-methods design, to ensure the most can be made of the wealth of data that results. In particular, combining-methods can become very complex when dealing with complex whole systems, aggravating challenges of cost and expertise requirements (given the only recent emergence of combined-research methodology, it remains difficult to find such expertise) and adding substantially to logistical problems. In addition, in adding qualitative research, the results may become less generalisable. Last, as indicated above, qualitative research, by its very nature, can change the intervention.

Summary

Combining qualitative research with the RCT constitutes a promising approach for CAM-intervention research. Pragmatically, qualitative research and the RCT should be combined so that the strengths of each method can overcome the weaknesses inherent in the other. The RCT is a superior design to assess intervention effectiveness while qualitative research is superior to explore meaning, context and process. Combined, qualitative research and the RCT constitute a rigorous research design that can achieve high internal, external and model validity.

Several recent and ongoing examples from the field have been utilised here to illustrate how combining methods can provide enhanced understanding of how an intervention works and in what context. Further, combining methods has provided the opportunity to explore the variety of physical, emotional and spiritual outcomes that CAM interventions offer to many patients. To date, however, most combined methods research has been sequential and not iterative, and much has not assessed the many varied processes and contextual factors that are essential to healing through CAM interventions. Both CAM intervention research and combined-methods research are still in their infancy.

An iterative, flexible whole systems research strategy appears to be the most relevant approach for the future of CAM intervention research. The multivariate nature of CAM interventions requires that they be approached in an iterative, integrated and flexible manner that considers qualitative and quantitative data at many points and with equal priority. No one research study can definitively answer whether and how an intervention may work. A programme of research is required that builds upon previous knowledge and learns from varied philosophical perspectives.

In the emerging field of whole systems research, however, there is no clear blueprint as how to best approach the important research questions of whether and how CAM interventions may work. Knowledge translation and knowledge transfer will thus be important so that we can learn from studies that are underway or have been completed. The whole systems strategy provides a comprehensive framework from which to approach CAM intervention research; however, the need for further conceptualising and operationalising is great.

Notes

1 The described limitations are not as pronounced when herbal preparations are being assessed.
2 The limitations of the RCT design for achieving model validity are outside the scope of this chapter. Refer to Verhoef et al. (2005) for a detailed discussion.

References

Adams, J., Sibbritt, D., Easthope, G. and Young, A. (2003) 'The profile of women who consult alternative health practitioners in Australia' *Medical Journal of Australia*, 179 (6): 297–300.
Alraek, T. and Baerheim, A. (2001) ' "An empty and happy feeling in the bladder . . .": health changes experienced by women after acupuncture for recurrent cystitis', *Complementary Therapies in Medicine*, 9 (4): 219–23.
—— (2003) 'The effect of prophylactic acupuncture treatment in women with recurrent

cystitis: kidney patients fared better', *Journal of Alternative and Complementary Medicine*, 9 (5): 651–8.

Barker, C. and Pistrang, N. (2005) 'Quality criteria under methodological pluralism: implications for conducting and evaluating research', *American Journal of Community Psychology*, 35 (3–4): 201–12.

Barnes, P., Powell-Griner, E., McFann, K. and Nahin, R. L. (2004) 'Complementary and alternative medicine use among adults: United States, 2002', *Advance Data*, 27 (343): 1–19.

Brazier, A., Mulkins, A. and Verhoef, M. (2006) 'Evaluating a yogic breathing and meditation intervention for individuals living with HIV/AIDS', *American Journal of Public Health*, 20 (3): 192–5.

Bryman, A. (2001) *Social Research Methods*, Oxford: Oxford University Press.

Buchanan, D. R. (1992) 'An uneasy alliance: combining qualitative and quantitative research methods', *Health Education Quarterly*, 19 (1): 117–35.

Cohen-Katz, J., Wiley, S., Capuano, T., Baker, D. M., Deitrick, L. and Shapiro, S. (2005) 'The effects of mindfulness-based stress reduction on nurse stress and burn-out: a qualitative and quantitative study, part III', *Holistic Nursing Practice*, 19 (2): 78–86.

Coyle, J. and Williams, B. (2000) 'An exploration of the epistemological intricacies of using qualitative data to develop a quantitative measure of user views of health care', *Journal of Advanced Nursing*, 31 (5): 1235–43.

Creswell, J. (2003) *Research Design: Qualitative, Quantitative and Mixed Methods Approaches*, Thousand Oaks, Calif.: Sage.

Greene, J. C., Caracelli, V. J. and Graham, W. F. (1989) 'Toward a conceptual frame-work for mixed-method evaluation designs', *Educational Evaluation and Policy Analysis*, 11 (3): 255–74.

Kligler, B. and Lee, R. (2004) *Integrative Medicine. Principles for Practice*, New York: McGraw-Hill.

Lewith, G. T., Walach, H. and Jonas, W. (2002) 'Balanced research strategies for complementary and alternative medicine', in G. T. Lewith, W. Jonas and H. Walach (eds) *Clinical Research in Complementary Therapies: Principles, Problems and Solutions*, Edinburgh: Churchill Livingstone, pp. 3–27.

Mehling, W. E., Hamel, K. A., Acree, M., Byl, N. and Hecht, F. M. (2005) 'Random-ised, controlled trial of breath therapy for patients with chronic low-back pain', *Alternative Therapies in Health and Medicine*, 11 (4): 44–52.

Morgan, D. L. (1998) 'Practical strategies for combining qualitative and quantitative methods: applications to health research', *Qualitative Health Research*, 8 (3): 362–76.

Morse, J. (1996) 'Is qualitative research complete?', *Qualitative Health Research*, 6 (1): 3–5.

Newman, I., Ridenour, C. S., Newman, C. and DeMarco, G. M. P. (2003) 'A typology of research purposes and its relationship to mixed methods', in A. Tashakkori and C. Teddlie (eds) *Handbook of Mixed Methods in Social and Behavioral Research*, Thousand Oaks, Calif.: Sage, pp. 167–88.

Patton, M. (1990) *Utilization Focused Evaluation*, Thousand Oaks, Calif.: Sage.

Polit, D. and Hungler, B. (1999) 'Integration of qualitative and quantitative designs', in D. Polit and C. T. Beck (eds) *Nursing Research: Principles and Methods*, Philidelphia, Pa.: Lippincott-Raven, pp. 273–86.

Ritenbaugh, C., Verhoef, M., Fleishman, S., Boon, H. and Leis, A. (2003) 'Whole systems research: a discipline for studying complementary and alternative medicine', *Alternative Therapies in Health and Medicine*, 9 (4): 32–6.

Sandelowski, M. (2000) 'Combining qualitative and quantitative sampling, data collection, and analysis techniques in mixed-methods studies', *Research in Nursing and Health*, 23 (3): 246–55.

Stange, K. (2004) 'Multimethod research', *Annals of Family Medicine*, 2 (1): 2–3.

Tashakkori, A. and Teddlie, C. (2003) *Handbook of Mixed Methods in Social and Behavioural Research*, Thousand Oaks, Calif.: Sage.

Verhoef, M. J. (2005) 'Placebo in qualitative studies: where is it hiding?', *Research Seminar on Complementary and Alternative Treatment*, Sommarøy, Norway, 15–16 March.

Verhoef, M., Casebeer, A. and Hilsden, R. (2002) 'Assessing efficacy of complementary medicine: adding qualitative research methods to the "Gold Standard" ', *Journal of Alternative and Complementary Medicine*, 8 (3): 275–81.

Verhoef, M., Lewith, G., Ritenbaugh, C., Boon, H., Fleishman, S. and Leis, A. (2005) 'Complementary and alternative medicine whole systems research: beyond identification of inadequacies of the RCT', *Complementary Therapies in Medicine*, 13 (3): 206–12.

Part II

Issues from the field

Chapter 6

Evidence and CAM research
Challenges and opportunities

Marc Cohen

Introduction: the need for evidence

With the increasing mainstreaming of CAM in all advanced societies (Tovey et al. 2004) it can be extremely difficult for medical administrators, politicians, practitioners and patients to know which therapies should be considered for any particular condition and which therapies are worthless or potentially dangerous. Government health-care funding is invariably limited and rarely provides sufficient resources to service all the health needs of a community. Politicians are therefore frequently faced with choices regarding the types of health care to fund and the types of research to support. Similarly, clinicians and patients must make decisions as to the most appropriate therapies to administer or receive. In order to help with these decisions, the use of evidence is vital; evidence can be a powerful clinical and political tool.

Evidence is also the cornerstone to developing a rigorous scientific approach to CAM and as the use and availability of CAM grows so too does the need to discuss and debate the notion of evidence and its place in making informed practice decisions. Nevertheless, collecting and interpreting evidence is not necessarily the same for CAM as it is for more conventional treatments, and there are specific challenges and opportunities facing CAM researchers and the broader CAM field in the attempt to provide and apply evidence. Furthermore, while evidence is extremely important, it is not the only consideration when it comes to making decisions about interventions affecting human health. There are many personal, social, cultural, economic, political and professional factors that impact on decision-making, many of which have specific implications for CAM (Tovey et al. 2004).

This chapter explores some of the debates regarding the role of evidence in relation to investigating CAM and examines a number of challenges associated with the evaluation and appropriation of evidence which currently face individual CAM researchers/practitioners and the broader CAM research community.

What is evidence?

In very simple terms the use of evidence to inform medical decision-making means applying knowledge and experience from the past to inform current practice with the aim of ensuring that this practice is more likely to do good than harm. In these terms, empirical evidence for different health-care practices has been accumulating since the beginnings of recorded history, and contemporary health professionals are currently inundated with information about evidence for a vast range of diverse health practices (Burgers et al. 2003).

As a result of increasing research activity, scientific evidence about CAM is now also accumulating from a number of sources. These sources include:

- in-vitro and laboratory studies looking at fundamental biological processes involved with therapies;
- animal studies conducted in both normal animals and animal models of disease;
- studies performed on humans that include anecdotal reports, individual case studies, case-control and cohort studies, randomised, double-blind, placebo-controlled trials of specific interventions for particular diseases;
- meta-analyses and systematic reviews of RCTs;
- epidemiological studies looking at disease patterns in large populations.

Evaluating and appropriating this evidence to guide clinical practice can be challenging; it can be difficult to understand the relevance of in-vitro or biochemical studies to clinical use, and the results of animal studies cannot always be extrapolated to humans. The complexity of applying evidence to clinical decision-making is compounded by the thousands of studies published every year with varying degrees of clinical relevance and methodological rigour. Furthermore, the results of studies are not always clear-cut, as there are often conflicting results, interpretations and ongoing controversies. Experts may also disagree about such basic issues as the most appropriate pain-management strategies for elderly patients (Chodosh 2001) or the existence of acupuncture points and meridians (Cho et al. 2002).

Evidence can be seen to exist in a hierarchy of forms, and the current system of academic endeavour and publishing has evolved in the attempt to expand our knowledge by providing access to the best available evidence upon which to make health and health-care decisions. This system of gathering and disseminating evidence includes an extensive international system of peer-reviewed literature that can be electronically searched, allowing authors and citations to be tracked and impact factors for journals to be calculated. There is also now an intricate system for cataloguing and systematically reviewing particular kinds of evidence through such organisations such as the Cochrane Collaboration (see Manheimer and Ezzo, Chapter 2, for a more detailed discussion of systematic reviews and CAM), and there are now guidelines for assessing scientific evidence such as those published by the Australian Government's National Health and Medical Research Council (NHMRC 2000). These guidelines classify evidence according to multiple dimensions including level, quality, statistical precision, effect size and relevance.

Regardless of such directives and guides, applying evidence in clinical practice can still be extremely complex. For example, there are many different types of research questions relating to CAM that can be addressed. These include questions such as whether a particular therapy works in theory (a question of efficacy) or is useful in clinical practice (a question of effectiveness) as well as whether the use of a therapy is safe and cost-effective. Furthermore, there is the quite separate question as to the mechanism of action by which a therapy actually works. It is common for evidence to suggest that a therapy is beneficial without knowing its mechanism of action. Conversely, the mechanism of action may be known but questions as to whether the therapy provides clinical benefit may remain unanswered.

It should be noted that the extent and quality of evidence for CAM treatments is often quite different to conventional medicine, as CAM research often proceeds in a different direction to conventional medical research. Research into new pharmaceutical compounds generally begins with laboratory or theoretical studies on the particular receptor or biochemical pathway to be targeted. Following such studies is then the development of specific molecules and the preclinical testing of these molecules in vitro and in vivo for toxicity, teratogenicity and mutagenicity (Steele et al. 1998). Drawing upon this early work, research then proceeds to Phase I clinical trials involving a small group of subjects in order to evaluate safety and appropriate dosage. This is then followed by Phase II and III trials to obtain further information on safety and efficacy and to provide comparison with other commonly used treatments. If these different phases of research yield successful results, the compound may then be registered and marketed and may be subject to Phase IV trials to gather information on its effect in various populations and to assess any side effects associated with long-term use. Completing all these phases of development often proves extremely expensive with the average cost of developing a marketable drug estimated to be around 800 million US dollars (DiMasi et al. 2003).

Research into CAM products and therapies often proceeds in a very different manner to that outlined above, with CAM often widely used in practice before any formal scientific research has been performed (Berman and Straus 2004, MacLennan et al. 2006). Formal scientific research, if it does occur, more often than not commences with RCTs in order to confirm or deny the effectiveness of treatment. From this initial work, research may then progress to the laboratory (including physiological, as well as animal and in-vitro studies) to determine the mechanisms underlying the effects of the treatment. Thus, while volumes of rigorous research are required to support the use of pharmaceuticals on the market, there is often little or no formal scientific research for the majority of CAM therapies in widespread use. Furthermore, the research that is performed into CAM does not necessarily represent what actually occurs in clinical practice (Vickers 1998) (for more detailed discussion of this point in relation to RCTs, see Pirotta, Chapter 4).

As a result of these circumstances there is often a conflict between research priorities and the way CAM is practised. Clinically focused research is based predominantly on statistical analysis and aims to produce results that can be applied to wider populations. The results of such research cannot provide specific information about an individual patient other than to suggest probabilities of different outcomes. Clinicians on the other hand, and particularly clinicians involved in CAM, focus on the individual patient for each consultation and take great care to account for the factors that a researcher may simply consider as 'confounding' (Cohen 2004). Moreover, researchers attempt to isolate the specific effects of a treatment by attempting to consider only a single treatment or a carefully prescribed combination of treatments through removing bias and the non-specific (placebo) effects of treatment. Meanwhile, a clinician will often utilise multiple treatments and may attempt to maximise non-specific effects to produce the best clinical outcome for a specific patient.

Employing evidence: towards a level playing field?

> As evidence emerges that some complementary medicines are effective, it becomes ethically impossible for the medical profession to ignore them.
>
> (AMA 2002)

While evidence is not the only consideration when making treatment decisions and research priorities are not always consistent with the approach of many CAM therapies, the accumulation and evaluation of evidence provides the basis for assessing CAM in the same terms as conventional medicine (Willis and White 2004). Thus evidence provides a level playing field by which any intervention can be judged and allows any therapy to be removed from its historical and philosophical basis and to be measured according to the common yardstick of the randomised controlled clinical trial (Institute of Medicine 2005); here the emphasis is upon *outcome* rather than explanation of therapy or treatment (Willis and White 2004). One potential advantage of this approach for CAM is that a treatment (regardless of origin) deserves serious consideration in mainstream practice if it has been successfully identified as safe and effective (Ernst 2003).

It has been conclusively demonstrated that a number of CAM therapies are at least as effective as comparable pharmaceutical preparations and often are safer and have fewer side effects (Ernst et al. 2001). Examples of such evidence-based CAM treatments include glucosamine compared to NSAIDs for osteoarthritis (Towheed et al. 2005), saw palmetto compared to the drug finasteride for benign prostatic hypertrophy (Wilt and MacDonald 2005) and St John's wort compared to tricyclic antidepressants or selective serotonin reuptake inhibitors (SSRIs) for mild to moderate depression (Linde et al. 2005). Despite this growing evidence base, the demonstration of evidence for CAM does not necessarily translate into mainstream acceptance and practice, and it appears that evidence is only a small part of the picture when it comes to identifying those therapies to be utilised – there remain powerful educational, administrative, economic and political factors that currently favour the use of pharmaceuticals.

More than evidence: the example of CAM for osteoarthritis in Australian practice

The use of CAM for osteoarthritis in the Australian context provides an excellent example of how safe and effective CAM therapies can remain underutilised.

The most common conventional treatment for osteoarthritis is the use of NSAIDs; however, while these drugs are in widespread use, they merely treat the pain of osteoarthritis and may in fact accelerate the course of the disease (Rashad and Hemingway 1989). They are also associated with gastrointestinal side effects as well as both renal and cardiac toxicity with significant associated morbidity and mortality, particularly in the elderly (Day and Roughead 1999). It is estimated that between 5 and 50 per cent of people have dyspepsia while taking an NSAID (Wolfe and Singh 1999), and in Australia alone it is estimated that there are 4,500 hospital admissions each year for serious gastrointestinal side effects due to NSAIDs with 10 per cent of these people dying directly as a consequence (Day and Roughead 1999). Furthermore, while the introduction of the COX-2 inhibitors may reduce the incidence of some gastrointestinal side effects in the short term, they may have similar effects on renal function and blood pressure (Group TAC-SICP 2002). It has even been suggested that the death rate due to NSAID-related cardiac failure may be more prevalent than NSAID-induced gastrointestinal side effects and that in Australia NSAID-induced cardiac failure contributes to as many as 8,000 hospital admissions and 800 deaths annually (Day and Roughead 1999). The recent voluntary worldwide recall of the Cox-2 inhibitor rofecoxib (vioxx) is a testimony of the potential dangers of these agents.

Nevertheless, NSAIDs remain in widespread use, and this places a considerable burden on society due to the direct cost of the drugs, the cost of the associated concomitant anti-ulcer medications, hospitalisations and deaths, not to mention the human cost in terms of associated morbidity and mortality. Any treatment that can replace or reduce the reliance on NSAID medication in the treatment of osteoarthritis would represent a significant advance, and there is mounting evidence that a range of CAMs may fulfil this role. Furthermore, while there are presently no curative therapies for osteo-arthritis, there is mounting evidence that CAM therapies such as glucosamine have the potential to not only address the symptoms but also to modify the underlying disease process (Towheed et al. 2005).

A recent study has reviewed the evidence for conventional treatments for osteoarthritis along with a limited number of CAM treatments and has compared them in terms of cost, safety and efficacy (Segal 2002). The results of this study were expressed in terms of Australian dollars per quality adjusted life year (QALY) with a low cost/QALY representing a cheap and highly effective and safe therapy and a high cost representing an expensive or an ineffective or dangerous therapy (Segal 2002). The study identified exercise programmes, self-management programmes and glucosamine as amongst the most cost-effective therapies with a cost/QALY of around 2,000–5,000 Australian dollars while the least cost-effective therapies were the non-specific NSAIDs at around 15,000 – infinity Australian dollars per QALY and the COX-2-specific inhibitors at around 33,000 – infinity Australian dollars per QALY. Other treatments such as knee-bracing and surgery had an estimated cost per QALY of between $5,000 and $10,000 (Segal 2002).

Despite the clear benefits of glucosamine over other treatments (including NSAIDS), the current Australian health-care environment favours the use of NSAIDS. The Government currently subsidises NSAIDS through the pharmaceutical benefits schedule (PBS) which provides tax-payer-funded subsidies for pharmaceutical drugs. Meanwhile, a 'CAM product' such as glucosamine does not receive a PBS subsidy while it does attract an added goods and services tax. This puts patients and practitioners in an invidious position. When faced with a typical elderly pensioner seeking pain relief for their osteoarthritis, a doctor can write a tax-payer-subsidised prescription for an NSAID that will cost the patient around 4.60 Australian dollars out of pocket for a month's supply yet expose them to potentially dangerous side effects and worsening of their condition. Conversely, the doctor can recommend the patient to purchase glucosamine which may provide greater clinical benefits yet will cost the patient more than three times the price of an NSAID.

It should be noted that the Australian Government does not accept responsibility for listing products on the PBS (Pharmaceutical Benefits Scheme 2005); instead it relies on submissions from industry that involve providing detailed evidence of the products' efficacy, safety and cost-effectiveness. While products such as glucosamine are not excluded from being eligible for PBS subsidies, no company to date has seen an economic advantage in listing such products on the PBS as there are significant associated administrative costs and the price provided to the company is often much lower than what would be recouped from direct sales. As such, the current Australian health-service delivery environment discriminates against CAM even in those cases where there is a strong evidence base. Perhaps what is needed is a complementary medicine benefits schedule (in addition to a PBS) that could facilitate the distribution of proven CAM products. Such a scheme does appear unlikely given the powerful vested interests in the current status quo which supports a pharmaceutical agenda.

Evidence is big business: difficulties for CAM research

Evidence for health-care treatments (whether CAM or conventional) is big business, and the current system of producing and reporting evidence is subject to many different interests including government and regulatory authorities, commercial interests such as the pharmaceutical and food industries, disease advocacy and consumer groups and the interests of individual researchers, editors and publishers. Perhaps the most powerful interests are those of the pharmaceutical industry as evidenced by the fact that in 2002 the combined profits for the top ten drug companies in the Fortune 500 were greater than those of all the other 490 companies combined (Angell 2004).

Just as evidence is important for the acceptance and utilisation of CAM, it is also important for the acceptance and utilisation of pharmaceuticals. The ability to produce and market drugs is totally dependent on having appropriate supporting evidence, and clinical trial results can dramatically influence the share price of companies whose products are being tested. As such, there are powerful incentives for drug companies to influence the design and conduct of trials as well as the content, publication and dissemination of their results.

As Marcia Angell, a former Editor-in-Chief of the *New England Journal of Medicine*, claims with a focus upon the US context,

> Over the past two decades the pharmaceutical industry has moved very far from its original high purpose of discovering and producing useful new drugs. Now primarily a marketing machine to sell drugs of dubious benefit, this industry uses its wealth and power to co-opt every institution that might stand in its way, including the US Congress, the FDA, academic medical centers, and the medical profession itself.
>
> (Angell 2004: 4)

While the conduct of research may be guided by methodological principles which aim to reduce bias and produce objective results, the selection of research projects is also open to bias. Ties between academia and pharmaceutical companies may not only lead to less research into the causes and mechanisms of disease (Angell 2000), but also less research into CAM.

The ability of a researcher to undertake an investigation more often than not rests upon attracting competitive funding, and investigators are often forced to undertake research commissioned and driven by particular funding bodies. This places CAM researchers at a distinct disadvantage: even after taking into account the recent moves in the USA and elsewhere to create dedicated funding for CAM research through bodies such as the National Centre for Complementary and Alternative Medicine (NCCAM), the funds available for CAM research are minimal (some might say negligible) compared to the money available for pharmaceutical research (Bensoussan and Lewith 2003, Ernst 1999).

Certainly, any research which is to be successfully completed requires considerable time, motivation and expertise from a team of people in addition to significant infrastructure and funding. This is generally more difficult to achieve for CAM than for pharmaceuticals due to there being far fewer researchers, institutes and funds to support CAM research than for more established medical research areas. Furthermore, much clinically focused CAM research that is currently undertaken is concerned with the use of product-related therapies (such as herbs and nutrients) which are underwritten by commercial interests as opposed to the use of therapies based on practitioner interventions (such as massage) where there are fewer commercial interests and fewer opportunities for research funding. There is also less research into the 'big questions' surrounding CAM, such as: What is the nature of 'life energy'? Do acupuncture meridians and points exist? How do placebos work? What is the relationship between the mind and the manifestation of health and disease? This is an unfortunate state of affairs as it remains likely that the greatest breakthroughs in our understanding about health and disease will come from exploring these and similar questions rather than merely confirming or denying the efficacy of different herbal or nutritional preparations in specific diseases.

The majority of existing CAM research appears to focus on the use of herbs, nutrients and other product-based therapies, yet, attracting funding for this type of research is also not without its difficulties. There is little incentive for companies to invest in research if their products cannot be patented, and CAM products do not usually contain unique patentable compounds. Unless a company has patented the production process, investment in research may provide equal benefit to competing companies who sell the same or similar products.

A further disincentive for the CAM industry to support research is the fact that CAM therapies do not require the same level of rigorous supporting evidence as pharmaceuticals before they can be marketed. In many countries such as the USA, CAM products are regulated as foods and do not require evidence of efficacy in order for them to be marketed (Cohen 2003). Even in countries such as Australia which have very strict CAM-product regulations, these products only require evidence of safety and quality and do not necessarily require research into their efficacy before sale (Australian Government Department of Health and Ageing 2005). Companies may deem it more effective to invest money into public-relations campaigns and advertising rather than invest in research that may potentially show that their best-selling products may be ineffective. In these circumstances, the appearance of an emotive case study about a CAM product on a television current-affairs programme may be considered a more cost-effective way of boosting sales than investment in research, which may have uncertain results.

The relative lack of funding for CAM research means that there are very few clinical research centres dedicated to exploring this field and few dedicated researchers with the necessary skills to perform high-quality CAM intervention research to assess efficacy. Most established research centres and experienced researchers are enticed to perform pharmaceutical research by the promise of lucrative grants and the potential for enormous profits. This leaves the pool of researchers available to perform work on CAM greatly diminished. Furthermore, successful CAM research requires the involvement of CAM practitioners who, despite a seemingly slow but sure growth in research capacity, are still more likely to be interested in clinical practice where they can enjoy a stable income and the satisfaction of patient contact (see Steinsbekk, Chapter 7, for a more detailed discussion of research-capacity-building among CAM practitioners).

Redefining CAM

Most clinically orientated CAM research is not actually research into CAM as practised but rather research into some of the 'tools of the trade' of CAM practitioners. Such research then acts to absorb aspects of CAM into mainstream medicine and can potentially lead to a 'takeover' whereby those CAM treatments found to be effective are monopolised by the medical community (Willis and White 2004). For example, there have been many RCTs on the use of single herbs for specific medical conditions. This has led to a growing evidence base for particular herbs and an increased utilisation of these herbs by the community and the mainstream medical profession. However, research into single herbs and their subsequent clinical use places herbs into a pharmaceutical model whereby they are matched to a diagnosis and used instead of a drug. This use of so-called 'green drugs' may be appropriate in cases where the herb has been shown to have demonstrated efficacy and safety, yet it does not necessarily represent the original CAM practice of herbal medicine. Herbalists rarely use single herbs, preferring to base their practice upon the extemporaneous compounding of different herbal preparations into concoctions designed to meet the needs of specific patients and their ailments at each presentation (Mills and Bone 2000).

Most CAM therapies attempt to be holistic in their approach, individualising treatments to the many factors that may influence their patients' health at each visit (Coulter 2004). Ancient systems of medicine such as TCM and Ayurvedic medicine, as well as the practice of Western herbal medicine, have sophisticated systems of categorising people according to different physiological and psychological characteristics which then form the basis for a highly individualised approach to therapy.

Meanwhile, in contrast, the task of the clinical researcher is often to minimise these factors and to standardise both patients and treatments so that fair comparisons can be produced. Accounting for individual differences – the basis for the *art* of medicine and the cornerstone of ancient medical wisdom – is difficult to incorporate in scientific trials. Despite the herbalists' practice of 'phytophenomics' (whereby herbal preparations are matched to a patient's appearance and which can be seen as a forerunner of the modern development of pharmaco-genomics promising to individualise drug therapy based on an individual's genetic profile [Evans and Relling 1999]), modern pharmaceutical science is yet to progress to a stage where drugs can be individualised for the specific needs of individual patients.

Another area where traditional practice can be seen to lead modern science is in the application of 'polychemical' medicine. While modern medicine generally discourages polypharmacy (Isenalumhe 1988), CAM practitioners are generally comfortable administering herbal preparations that contain numerous different compounds that may act in synergy to produce a desired therapeutic effect. Thus there may be much to be gained from the scientific study of traditions, such as those of Chinese medicine, which have developed principles to guide the preparation of herbal formulas whereby one herb may provide the main desired activity while others will be included to improve bioavailability and tissue selectivity or to reduce side effects (Lee 2000).

Some effective treatments will never have evidence

With so much current emphasis placed on the use of evidence, it is important to recognise that a lack of evidence for a particular effect does *not* mean there is evidence for a lack of effect. No evidence is not the same as negative evidence; it simply means that the research has not yet been done. It is also important to recognise that due to financial, methodological or logistical constraints, some treatments will *never* have evidence and that this does not necessarily mean that the treatment is ineffective or worthless.

A good example of a treatment that is unlikely to ever have rigorous supporting evidence is the treatment of an acute asthma attack with acupuncture which involves the deep insertion of an acupuncture needle into the suprasternal notch (the hollow at the base of the neck). Anecdotal reports suggest that this procedure is effective and potentially life-saving, yet there are a number of factors that make it unlikely that this treatment will ever be subject to a rigorous randomised controlled study. First, a study into this treatment is unlikely to be funded as there is no product involved and no financial incentive for any commercial body to obtain advantage from the procedure. Acupuncture needles are very inexpensive and their use in this specific situation would not result in any significant increased sales. Second, this procedure is invasive and possesses significant inherent risk and it would be extremely difficult to obtain approval from a human-ethics committee for such a study. Third, it would be very difficult to obtain informed consent from subjects to participate in such a study as consent would need to be obtained while subjects were experiencing a distressing and potentially life-threatening event. Finally, it would be difficult to find an experienced acupuncturist to participate in such a trial with access to the necessary patients along with the institutional support and facilities necessary to perform the research.

Factors to consider when making treatment decisions

Evidence is only one consideration, albeit a key one, when making decisions about health care. Other factors include the personal preferences of both the practitioner and the patient, the range of possible alternatives, the associated costs and risks versus the potential benefits of a proposed treatment, as well as aspects of expedience such as availability, accessibility and immediacy of treatment.

It may be comforting to think that all treatment decisions are based on rational principles yet this is certainly not the case. Every decision about a therapeutic intervention must also include acknowledgement of personal preferences. Patients, practitioners and researchers all bring their own unique personal, ideological, religious, ethical, cultural, educational and philosophical biases that influence the types of treatments considered appropriate to either receive, practise or research. These biases may be particularly prominent in the case of CAM. CAM therapies are often aligned (or claim alignment) with philosophies or ideologies that have strong community support such as environmentalism, spiritualism and vitalism (Coulter 2004), and individuals may be drawn to particular therapies based not on evidence of efficacy but on other personal considerations that they find hard to articulate and explicable only to themselves.

While personal preference may defy rational explanation and may even conflict with the best available evidence, informed consent and respect for patient autonomy are amongst the highest ethical principles in medicine (Meisel 1996). Practitioners must respect the rights of their patients to make their own informed decisions as to the type of health care they wish to receive and to either refuse or accept any treatment offered. It also follows that all patients have a responsibility to become more informed and to be active participants in the decision-making process. This is certainly happening with the use of CAM which is generally patient- rather than practitioner-driven (Edlin 2003). However, true informed consent is difficult to achieve as it is rare for either patients or practitioners to have access to all relevant information.

The requirement for informed consent further places an ethical (and possibly legal) obligation upon practitioners to fully inform their patients about the range of possible treatments they offer and the associated risks of such treatments in addition to declaring their own practice limitations and biases. It also places responsibility on orthodox medical practitioners to know about, or at least have readily accessible resources available regarding, common CAM therapies that may impact on any prescribed orthodox treatments. Becoming informed about different health-care options generally means becoming aware of the strengths and weaknesses of the available scientific evidence. This includes reviewing the evidence of safety and efficacy for the therapy under consideration as well as understanding the inherent limitations of the available evidence and relevance to a specific situation. In addition to reviewing the evidence for a particular therapy there may be a range of therapeutic alternatives that may be used together or in isolation. Thus, it may be necessary to review the evidence for a number of different therapies and to weigh the evidence for one treatment against that for others.

The weighing-up of evidence involves not only an assessment of quality but also of costs and risks versus potential benefits. A treatment which is risky or comes at high cost generally needs to be balanced by a large potential benefit before it is utilised, whereas a treatment that poses little risk and has a low cost may be used even if the potential benefits are not so pronounced. In this analysis, CAM interventions are often looked on favourably, for although there may not be conclusive evidence of their effectiveness, there is often a long history of practical experience suggesting relative safety of use. Unfortunately, the same cannot often be said of many pharmaceutical or surgical interventions which often have the potential for serious adverse effects – a feature providing an additional driving force in the increasing utilisation of CAM (Siahpush 1998).

A further consideration when deciding on a therapeutic option is expedience. In order to utilise a particular treatment, the treatment must be available for use and readily accessible to the intended individual. If a particular therapy is appropriate but unavailable due to government regulations or inaccessible due to financial, geographical, logistic or other restrictions, then this must be taken into consideration. Furthermore, the timing and immediacy of treatment needs to be considered. Treatment received at the roadside or at a country clinic may be considerably different to treatment received at a tertiary teaching hospital. If a condition demands urgent treatment then the range of potential treatments is naturally limited to those that are immediately available whereas less urgent conditions may wait until a wider range of treatments can be accessed. Again, this influences the utilisation of CAM which is not commonly available in hospital emergency departments and less frequently utilised for acute and emergency cases than for chronic illnesses. Furthermore, most CAM therapies are not yet widely available and successful CAM practitioners often have long waiting lists, making it difficult for patients to access them for acute conditions.

The principles described above apply across all therapeutic modalities and should be applied to considerations of both conventional and complementary therapies. Furthermore, it is clear that of all the factors that must be considered when making treatment choices, individual factors are at least as important as the scientific evidence. Evidence, however, does play a special role as it represents the accumulated wisdom and experience of humanity and is being continually updated and refined as our collective experience expands. As such, it is clear that medical decision-making needs to be informed by the best available evidence. This simple premise has led to the principles of evidence-based medicine (EBM) described by Sackett et al. as 'the conscientious, explicit, and judicious use of current best evidence in making decisions about the care of individual patients' (Sackett et al. 1996). As Sackett et al. go on to explain:

> The practice of evidence based medicine means integrating individual clinical expertise with the best available external clinical evidence from systematic research. By individual clinical expertise we mean the proficiency and judgment that individual clinicians acquire through clinical experience and clinical practice. Increased expertise is reflected in many ways, but especially in more effective and efficient diagnosis and in the more thoughtful identification and compassionate use of individual patients' predicaments, rights, and preferences in making clinical decisions about their care.
>
> (Sackett 1996: 72)

Sackett acknowledges that for most practical treatment decisions, conclusive evidence simply does not as yet exist and that best available evidence may be clinical experience or anecdotal reports (Sackett et al. 1996). It thereby follows that CAM treatments, which often have a much longer history of use than conventional medicine, may be the most appropriate treatment for a range of conditions. Nevertheless, as discussed earlier, it is presumptuous to assume that evidence for a treatment necessarily leads to that treatment being adopted in practice.

Summary

The consideration of evidence provides a basis for making rational treatment decisions, and the accumulation of evidence provides enhanced respectability for CAM. Evidence offers a consistent basis for considering CAM treatments alongside conventional therapies. As this chapter has illustrated, there are many potential barriers to the accumulation and appropriation of evidence for CAM. Nevertheless, it would seem that the challenge facing medicine has to some extent only just begun. Consideration of the broad topic of evidence with regard to CAM helps reflect upon the relationship between evidence, research and medical practice more generally. While questions regarding evidence and its role in influencing treatment choice are central to researching and assessing CAM, these are not simply CAM questions but may yet prove to be the basis for a transformation of the biomedical paradigm and conventional medical practice.

References

AMA (2002) *AMA Position Statement Complementary Medicine*, Sydney: Australian Medical Association.

Angell, M. (2000) 'Is academic medicine for sale?' *New England Journal of Medicine*, 342: 1516–18.

—— (2004) *The Truth about Drug Companies*, New York: Random House.

Australian Government Department of Health and Ageing, Therapeutic Goods Administration (2005) *Australian Regulatory Guidelines for Complementary Medicines*, Sydney: ARGCM.

Bensoussan, A. and Lewith, G. T. (2003) 'Complementary medicine research in Australia: a strategy for the future', *Medical Journal of Australia*, 181 (6): 331–3.

Berman, J. D. and Straus, S. E. (2004) 'Implementing a research agenda for complementary and alternative medicine', *Annual Reviews of Medicine*, 55: 239–54.

British Medical Association (1993) *Complementary Medicine: New Approaches to Good Practice*, Oxford: Oxford University Press.

Burgers, J. S., Grol, R., Klanzinga, N. S., Mäkelä, M. and Zaat, J. (2003) 'Towards evidence-based clinical practice: an international survey of 18 clinical guideline programmes', *International Journal for Quality in Health Care*, 15 (1): 31–45.

Cho, Z. H., Oleson, T. D., Alimi, D., Niemtzow, R. C. (2002) 'Acupuncture: the search for biologic evidence with functional magnetic resonance imaging and positron emission tomography techniques', *Journal of Alternative and Complementary Medicine*, 8 (4): 399–401.

Chodosh, J., Ferrell, B. A., Shekelle, P. G., Wenger, N. S. (2001) 'Quality indicators for pain management in vulnerable elders', *Annals of Internal Medicine*, 135 (8): 731–5.

Cohen, M.H. (2003) 'Complementary and integrative medical therapies, the FDA, and the NIH: definition and regulation', *Dermatologic Therapy*, 16: 77.

—— (2004) 'Negotiating integrative medicine: a framework for provider–patient conversations', *Negotiation Journal*, 20: 409.

Committee, P.B.A. (2005) *PBS Medicine List*.

Coulter, I. (2004) 'Integration and paradigm clash: the practical difficulties of integrative medicine', in P. Tovey, G. Easthope and J. Adams (eds) *The Mainstreaming of Complementary and Alternative Medicine: Studies in Social Context*, London: Routledge.

Day, R. R. and Roughead, E. E. (1999) 'Towards the safer use of non-steroidal antiinflammatory drugs', *Journal of Quality Practice*, 19 (1): 51–3.

DiMasi, J. A., Hansen, R. W. and Grabowski, K.G. (2003) 'The price of innovation: new estimates of drug development costs', *Journal of Health Economics*, 22: 151–85.

Edlin, M. (2003) 'Demand for CAM grows, but belongs in a separate benefit category', *Managed Health Care Executive*, 13 (6), 38–9.

Ernst, E. (1999) 'Funding research into complementary medicine: the situation in Britain', *Complementary Therapies in Medicine*, 7 (4): 250–3.

—— (2003) 'Complementary medicine: where is the evidence?', *Journal of Family Practice*, 52 (8): 630–4.

Ernst, E., Pittler, M. H., Stevinson, C., White, A. R. and Eisenberg, D. (2001) *The Desktop Guide to Complementary and Alternative Medicine*, Edinburgh: Mosby.

Evans, W. E. and Relling, M. V. (1999) 'Pharmacogenomics: translating functional genomics into rational therapeutics', *Science*, 286 (5439): 487–91.

Group, TAC-SICP (2002) 'Considerations for the safe prescribing and use of COX–2-specific inhibitors', *Medical Journal of Australia*, 176: 328–31.

Institute of Medicine (2005) *Complementary and Alternative Medicine in the United States*, Washington, DC: Academy Press.

Isenalumhe, A. E. (1988) 'Polypharmacy: its cost burden and barrier to medical care in a drug-oriented health care system', *International Journal of Health Services*, 18 (2): 335–42.

Kotsirilos, V. (2005) 'Complementary and alternative medicine. Part 2: evidence and implications for general practitioners', *Australian Family Physician*, 34 (8): 689–91.

Lee, K. H. (2000) 'Research and future trends in the pharmaceutical development of medicinal herbs from Chinese medicine', *Public Health Nutrition*, 3 (4a): 515–22.

Linde K. M. C., Berner M. and Egger, M. (2005) 'St John's Wort for depression', *The Cochrane Database of Systematic Reviews, (4)*.

MacLennan, A. H., Myers, S. P. and Taylor, A. W. (2006) 'The continuing cost of complementary and alternative medicine in South Australia: costs and beliefs in 2004', *Medical Journal of Australia*, 184 (1): 27–31.

Meisel, A. K. M. (1996) 'Legal and ethical myths about informed consent', *Archives of Internal Medicine*, 156 (22): 2521–6.

Mills, S. and Bone, K. (2000) *Principles and Practice of Phytotherapy*, London: Churchill Livingstone.

National Centre for Complementary and Alternative Medicine (2005) *Overview: What NCCAM Funds*, Bethesda, Md.: National Institutes of Health.

National Health and Medical Research Council (2000) *How to Use the Evidence: Assessment and Application of Scientific Evidence*, Canberra: NHMRC.

Rashad, S. R. P. and Hemingway A. (1989) 'Effect of nonsteroidal anti-inflammatory drugs on the course of osteoarthritis', *Lancet*, 2 (8662): 519–22.

Royal Australian College of General Practitioners and Australian as Integrative Medicine Association (2005) *RACGP/AIMA Joint Position Statement on Complementary Medicine*, Melbourne: RACGP-AIMA.

Sackett, D., Gray, W. M., Haynes, R. B., Richardson, W. S. (1996) 'Evidence based medicine: what it is and what it isn't', *British Medical Journal*, 312 (7023): 71–2.

Segal, L. (2002) *'Priority Setting in Osteoarthritis'*, Natural Healthcare Summit, Sydney, September.

Siahpush, M. (1998) 'Postmodern values, dissatisfaction with conventional medicine and popularity of alternative therapies', *Journal of Sociology*, 34 (1): 58–70.

Steele, V. E., Boone, C. W., Lubet, R. A., Crowell, J. A., Holmes, C. A., Sigman, C. C. and Kelloff, G. J. (1998) 'Preclinical drug development paradigms for chemopreventives', *Hematology/Oncology Clinics of North America*, 12 (5): 943–61, v–vi.

Tovey, P., Easthope, G. and Adams, J. (2004) (eds) *The Mainstreaming of Complementary and Alternative Medicine: Studies in Social Context*, London: Routledge.

Towheed, T. E., Anastassiades, T. P., Shea, B., Houpt, J., Robinson, V., Hochberg, M. C. and Wells, G. (2005) 'Glucosamine therapy for treating osteoarthritis', *The Cochrane Database of Systematic Reviews*, 4.

Vickers, A. (1998) 'Bibliometric analysis of randomized trials in complementary medicine', *Complementary Therapies in Medicine*, 6 (4): 185–9.

Willis, E. and White, K. (2004) 'Evidence-based medicine and CAM', in P. Tovey, G. Easthope and J. Adams (eds) *The Mainstreaming of Complementary and Alternative Medicine: Studies in Social Context*. London: Routledge, pp. 49–63.

Wilt, T. I. A. and MacDonald, R. (2005) 'Serenoa repens for benign prostatic hyperplasia', *The Cochrane Database of Systematic Reviews*, 4.

Wolfe, M. L. and Singh, G. (1999) 'Gastrointestinal toxicity of non-steroidal anti-inflammatory drugs', *New England Journal of Medicine*, 340 (24): 1888–99.

Chapter 7

The practitioner as researcher

Research capacity-building within the ranks of CAM

Aslak Steinsbekk

Introduction

In the course of their clinical practice, CAM therapists, like all types of health practitioners, encounter results that provide insight and clues to treating symptoms and disease. There are many examples of patients who experience and report positive reactions to their ongoing CAM treatment, and a practitioner devoted to the well-being of the community will understandably wish to inform other practitioners of such experiences and help extend relief to other patients.

On a broader level, it is also the case that a traditionally marginalised field such as CAM can often lack the empirical investigation or interest in the specific treatment or therapy attributed to other more conventional medicines (Lewith et al. 2003). This too can be a motivating factor for some CAM practitioners looking to design and conduct research themselves. Despite the growing focus upon CAM by the research community (Barnes et al. 1996, Bensoussan and Lewith 2004, Bondurant and Sox 2005, Raschetti et al. 2005), it is still the case that many treatments have not been tested for efficacy (Kotsirilos 2005). Faced with these somewhat frustrating circumstances and the often-noted call from the medical profession and media to produce the evidence for their therapeutic claims (Angell and Kassirer 1998, Kinsel and Straus 2003), CAM practitioners may quite understandably set out to address such research gaps themselves. Furthermore, their research involvement can also be an excellent complement to practice, providing a reflexivity that is beneficial to patient care (McLeod 1999, Zick and Benn 2004), and, on a broader level, may be conceptualised as one possible strategy for advancing the professional authority and status of the wider grouping of CAM providers.

CAM has been identified as a popular treatment choice in numerous countries (Harris and Rees 2000). For example, research exploring CAM in Scandinavian countries has identified 34 per cent CAM use in Norway, 45 per cent in Denmark and 49 per cent in Stockholm (Hanssen et al. 2005). Yet, we still know relatively little about what is actually done in clinical practice and CAM practitioners do have an important contribution to make to research investigating this and related topics.

Nevertheless, while practitioners' experiences and reported results form an interesting component of practice, they also require a systematic and well-prepared approach in order to gain an evidence-base research status and be more widely accepted within both the research and practice communities. It is important to acknowledge that the belief that research and practice necessarily draw upon similar skills is highly questionable (McIvor 1995), and it is equally important for CAM practitioners to understand the scientific research process as it is for researchers (who are not also practitioners) to engage with practice realities and needs (Zick and Benn 2004).

This chapter explores some of the key issues facing those CAM practitioners interested in initiating or advancing their research involvement in their own particular field of practice. A clinical background and perspective can bring both limits and advantages for conducting health research. While knowledge of the therapy and direct clinical experience can be important aids in designing and conducting CAM research projects, the skills and knowledge necessary to complete successful investigations are not always necessarily possessed by, or readily available to, CAM practitioners. This chapter addresses a selection of practical and methodological issues which have been highlighted through my own experience and which require attention in this particular type of research.

CAM practitioners can obviously develop interests and skills in a large range of research areas and approaches, and it is beyond the scope of this chapter to explore all possible perspectives and topics available. Here discussion is restricted primarily to research of *direct* relevance to aspects of clinical practice, investigation based upon different aims and exploring quite distinct topics (for example, social-science and health-services research that may examine the professional status and role of CAM practitioners) is acknowledged but not given priority here. The focus of this chapter, drawing extensively upon my own personal experience of CAM practice and research development, fits comfortably with the clinical focus and interest of a large number of CAM practitioners.

Attention is also partly concentrated upon the case study of research-development strategy as it pertains to homeopathy in Norway over the past decade. This case study acts as a useful vehicle for illustrating a range of issues facing both individual practitioners and the CAM practitioner community more generally. However, it should be noted that the issues and themes raised in this discussion are, in most cases, of relevance to practitioners of other CAM as well as those who may be practising CAM in other countries and who are also looking to become directly involved in research. Before moving on to discuss the challenges and opportunities facing individual practitioners who conduct research, this chapter first introduces a recent national strategy for developing insider CAM research within Norway and explores the core tenets of this model for practitioner research.

CAM practitioner-researcher development: drawing upon the Norwegian experience

Research capacity-building is not only the concern and responsibility of individual practitioners. Health research organisations, CAM research and practice organisations and CAM-practitioner representative bodies must also play an important role. Unfortunately, this is not always the case. For example, many CAM bodies representing therapists do not as yet dedicate adequate focus or funding to developing research in their therapy (Lewith and Holgate 2000, Wilder and Ernst 2003), and CAM research capacity-building has, to date, been largely ad hoc and lacking in sustained disciplinary debate or analysis (Andrews 2006).

Nevertheless, a number of schemes, programmes and strategies have emerged for enhancing research skills and output from amongst the ranks of CAM practitioners. In Canada, mentoring programmes have been introduced as a means of enabling multidisciplinary collaboration between academic CAM researchers and practitioners and promoting opportunities for developing research literacy and capacity amongst CAM practitioners (Leung et al. 2005). Similarly, a recent project grant partnership program run by the NCCAM in the USA aims to increase the quality and quantity of research content in the curricula at CAM institutions where CAM practitioners are trained (NCCAM 2004).

Similarly, the Norwegian Research Council (NRC) has been facilitating a politically initiated research programme for CAM since 1992 (Norges Offentlige Utredninger 1998). This programme has involved input from relevant CAM-practitioner representative bodies in the area of homeopathy, acupuncture, chiropractic, anthroposophical medicine and holistic health. Prior to the NRC programme there was very little CAM research in Norway with the few studies conducted being predominantly small-scale pilot work. These early studies met with ethical and financial difficulties. One example was a pilot study on the effect of homeopathic treatment for lower urinary tract infection which recruited twenty women in what became an observational study (Straumsheim 1990). This investigation did not progress beyond this initial pilot stage due to difficulties attracting additional funds as well as problems with ethical approval (this concerned the argument that no patient could be denied the best available treatment, antibiotics).

In the early days of the programme, the NRC provided mostly small grants (ranging from the equivalent of approximately 2,000 to 20,000 pounds sterling). As a result of this initial programme policy, a number of CAM practitioners received research funding that allowed them to develop protocols or to conduct studies alongside their clinical practice. Very few of these recipients had any prior research experience and the programme also initiated short courses in research methodology to help nurture research development from within the clinical ranks of CAM.

Although successful in encouraging practitioners to embrace research projects, this early funding was frequently too limited to encourage in-depth research education for practitioners. Based on the experience gained in these first few years, an evaluation was undertaken to consolidate the programme and to identify future needs. The research group of the Norwegian homeo-pathic society (Norske Homeopaters Landsforbund, NHL) published a strat-egy on the development of homeopathic research in Norway based on this evaluation (NHL 1997). The NHL strategy, which is partly presented below, illustrates some of the challenges facing the CAM field in encouraging practi-tioners to engage in research activity. In particular, it highlights the need to focus upon two distinct and parallel challenges: how to build on the core features of everyday CAM practice to develop a research agenda while, at the same time, fostering research competence amongst practitioners.

The three main objectives of the NHL strategy were: educating practitioners as researchers, encouraging organised data collection and establishing a research centre and fostering research networks. These three objectives will now be discussed in turn in more detail below.

Educating practitioners as researchers

A prime objective of the NHL strategy was to educate homeopaths as researchers (NHL 1997), the reasoning behind this being twofold. First, it was assumed that in order to develop homeopathy research, investigators needed to be qualified homeopaths with clinical experience. This was seen as essential to the development of high-quality research in homeopathy, the vision was to produce homeopaths with enough knowledge of research to be principal investigators and field leaders.

In addition, the difficulty for practitioners to collaborate with experienced researchers without having some personal grounding in research and methods was acknowledged in the NHL report. This raises an issue essential to the research capacity-building endeavours in any field of CAM. It is important that practitioners collaborating and working alongside researchers (who may not have a clinical training) provide more than just practice-based input and advice. If the development of research capacity from within prac-titioner ranks is a real goal for CAM, and if practitioners do not wish to be sidelined in any future research programmes, it is essential that practitioners themselves gain hands-on experience and transferable skills in all stages of the research process. As we will see later in this chapter, this issue is inextric-ably linked to the power relations amongst members of the multidisciplinary research team.

Another issue related to practitioner research training and highlighted by the NHL report relates to the fact that the vast majority of CAM therapists in Norway (including homeopaths) do not have an academic education (a situation not dissimilar to that for many CAM practitioners worldwide). As such, in order to follow the conventional career path of an academic researcher (that is, to complete a doctoral degree), a CAM practitioner will often first require full undergraduate academic training. Both the extensive period of learning required and the demand of finding time on a week-to-week basis to undertake such academic scholarship while also practising and earning a living are conceivably major challenges facing the majority of CAM practitioners looking to break into the world of research.

It can often prove difficult to keep pace with the fast-changing research literature while maintaining a busy patient load, especially given the lack of research training currently provided within CAM education (NCCAM 2004) and the fact that the research literacy of CAM practitioners, like that for other health-care delivery groups, leaves room for improvement (Leung et al. 2005). The added demands on a practitioner moving beyond reading research findings to actively training in methodology and research design can prove extremely testing, and in some cases may conceivably constitute a threat to the smooth operation of a clinical practice.

Encouraging organised data collection

The second objective of the NHL strategy, to 'conduct organised data collection in homeopathic practice' (NHL 1997: 10), was in response to the identification that a lack of knowledge and appreciation of clinical practice can make the planning of trials difficult. Addressing issues such as the appropriate type of patients/conditions to include, the appropriate treatments to administer and the expected outcomes, often relies more upon guesswork than informed decision-making. Organised data collection on behalf of practitioners can help overcome some of these difficulties by helping ensure a closer fit between research and the realities of clinical practice.

Documenting aspects of clinical practice through practitioner-based research development is also important for identifying an appropriate role for different types of CAM in the health market. Knowledge of the clinical strengths of different therapies provides useful guides for directing patients to relevant treatments, an issue highlighted with the move towards medical pluralism (Goldstein 2002) and the increasing number and range of CAM practitioners now available in most advanced societies (Tovey et al. 2004). As CAM becomes available in an increasing number of settings and is practised by a growing number of health professionals (in addition to CAM practitioners this includes GPs [Adams 2004, Botting and Cook 2000], nurses [Hunt et al. 2004], midwives [Tiran in press] and others), the possible styles of CAM practice are also increased. Again, this stresses the central role of

CAM practitioners in helping guide the agenda for research and thereby the possible practice directives that may result from such research.

The CAM practitioner-researcher is frequently faced with the need to prioritise what sort of research project to initiate. While there are many personal and political considerations, the decision regarding the focus and mode of research is usually heavily influenced by the need to gain funds, this means sometimes compromising the research adventure to reflect interests beyond that of the individual therapist.

From the point of view of a CAM researcher who is a practitioner in the field, it is often anticipated by other CAM practitioners that one engages in research in order to prove the value of the therapy – an understandable expectation given the marginalised status of CAM in the health-care arena – and it can be difficult to withstand such peer pressure without good counterargument and justification.

One justification for not restricting research focus purely upon the issue of efficacy is the need to place CAM research questions within the wider context of stakeholder perspectives. The development of research in CAM has to take into consideration that many CAM therapies and products are already frequently used by patients (Barnes et al. 2004, Eisenberg et al. 1998) and are also either a new or established part of state health services (such as homeopathy in the UK National Health Service (NHS)). As such, it is important to acknowledge that while different stakeholders may share both a common desire for research development and often a large body of research interest, there are different parties with particular and distinct research foci and priorities.

For example, from a governmental/regulatory view, it may be important to collect data that has direct impact on the provision and organisation of health-care services (Casey et al. in press, Giannelli et al. 2004). And this may be a focus not necessarily perceived as core or even helpful by others in the field (Ernst 2005).

Most efficacy research done on CAM therapies has used methodology developed to ensure a new drug does not receive authority approval before being proven safe and effective (Phase I–V, where Phase III is the double-blind RCT). This approach is highly valid in CAM research, but as many CAM therapies are already established therapies (sometimes with relatively early origins and long traditions of use), it is obvious that this approach cannot be conducted in isolation. One possible counter to such a restricted research focus is the use of an integrated structure of CAM research-building (Fonnebo 2003).

The starting point for this strategy is to produce data on the prevalence and features of therapy use in a community/country (for example, examining who is using CAM for which conditions and the motivation of users). Building upon this work, the next level consists of assuring the safety of everyday provision of the therapy in practice. Following on from this safety-assurance research is the examination of the effectiveness of the everyday practice of the therapy. A fourth level involves examining the efficacy of the specific components of the therapy (for example, the effect of a single intervention such as a drug or needle), and the final level of the structure is research investigating the mechanism of action of the intervention in the body.

Establishing a research centre and fostering networks

The third objective of the NHL strategy was to help foster networks *between* practitioner-researchers and to establish a research centre where they could meet and work. This policy highlights and addresses two main concerns in CAM research capacity-building. Many CAM practitioners can face isolation in their research adventure due to a lack of integration within a wider support network. Given their own practice time demands and the low numbers of research-active practitioners, it can often prove difficult to locate a colleague able to share and critique research ideas and more difficult still to identify a colleague conveniently positioned and qualified to conduct collaborative projects. This is partly the result of homeopaths' and CAM practitioners' traditional locations outside the university system, although this is slowly changing with the introduction of CAM research centres at some universities worldwide (examples being the Australian Centre for Complementary Medicine Education and Research at the University of Queensland and Southern Cross University, Australia, the Complementary Medicine Research Unit at the University of Exeter and Plymouth, England and the National Centre for Research in Complementary and Alternative Medicine at the University of Tromsø, Norway).

The isolation from research activity is also partly the result of the practice location of the CAM practitioner. While some CAM practitioners may establish informal referrals with conventional medical practitioners (Adams and Tovey 2000, Andrews 2004) and others may work in multidisciplinary teams based in one medical site (Coulter and Willis 2004, Hsiao et al. in press), the vast majority work as small private businesses (either in solo or with other CAM practitioners), an environment where economic survival is not necessarily conducive to research-building. Without a designated hub where practitioners can meet, share ideas and draw upon centrally provided research resources, some therapists find a parallel research career simply too demanding on their personal finances.

Local and often ad-hoc practitioner networks can act as avenues for practitioner development, but they are limited both by their reach and often unsystematic approach to information-sharing. Meanwhile, a CAM practitioner-based research programme as envisaged by the NHL strategy helps provide some of the depth, richness and quality of evidence lacking from less formal and structured networks.

As this selective overview of the NHL strategy and its objectives help to illustrate, a number of important issues face both the general development of practitioner research in CAM and individual CAM practitioners wishing to follow a research career. Before concluding this chapter, an additional challenge facing CAM practitioner-researchers is first discussed.

Working in a multidisciplinary team: difficulties of collaborative research

It is a great asset for all early-stage researchers to have contact and interaction with those more established in the field. As mentioned earlier, there is often a lack of research training in CAM education, and it is often essential that the practitioner looking to undertake research will require the initial help and guidance of a more experienced academic researcher. As a result, the majority of CAM research that does currently include practitioner input is housed within multidisciplinary teams (for example, see Casey et al. in press). However, while this team approach may be borne out of necessity, we do also need to critically appraise this model of research activity and consider potential problems: does a CAM practitioner plus an academic researcher make a suitable team for CAM research?

One potential problem with this team approach relates to the time required to learn and enhance essential research skills. The CAM practitioner might seek to avoid the intense and extensive research training initially involved in project development, and it may be tempting to sidestep this issue by abdicating responsibility for these early design issues to the skilled and experienced researcher. This situation obviously has serious implications for the research capacity-building within CAM ranks and ultimately can lead to the somewhat piecemeal and fringe input of practitioners within the research process.

Ideally, practitioner-researcher collaborations should involve a true sharing of skills and knowledge, the CAM practitioner providing and sharing knowledge and insight relating to aspects of practice while the academic researcher applies and shares their expertise in methodology and design. Unfortunately, it is all too easy to fall into traditional disciplinary roles and divisions of labour and this can lead to challenges in research design.

One outcome of this situation is that the therapy under investigation may be oversimplified and modified to meet methodological requirements. There are numerous trials where the CAM therapy has been simplified in order to match the requirements of the research design rather than being tailored to the specifics of the therapy (Mathie 2003). The result is that while CAM practitioners reading the final publication may not recognise the intervention (therapy) described as that used in daily practice, the trial nonetheless does often score highly in terms of methodological rigour.

A trial undertaken in Norway on homeopathic treatment for tooth extraction (Lokken et al. 1995) provides a good example of this tension in multidisciplinary CAM research. In the study, two wisdom teeth were extracted from each participant using a cross-over design where the participants received both the intervention (e.g., pain killer) and the control treatment (placebo) in random order. This trial has, correctly, been assigned very high methodological scores in review articles and meta-analyses (Linde et al. 1997) and the model has been used several times since to test the effect of various conventional interventions on signs and symptoms associated with soft tissue and bone injury.

This model was used to test the specific effects of individually prescribed homeopathic remedies in D-30 potency, namely arnica, hypericum, staphisagria, ledum, phosphorus and plantago. The homeopaths involved in the study found it difficult to choose the most appropriate homeopathic medicine as there were few identifiable individual symptoms (this probably explains why arnica – frequently used on any form of bruises – was identified as by far the most frequently prescribed medicine). This design is potentially problematic. Homeopathic practice in Norway mainly consists of treating chronic conditions (Steinsbekk and Fonnebo 2003). Patients do not refer directly from the dentist to the homeopath in order to receive treatment for any complaint that might arise in dental surgery. Moreover, there are few homeopaths in Norway who regularly treat patients following tooth extraction. So, even if the homeopaths participating in the study are suitably qualified and trained, they do not necessarily have experience in treating the exact patient group under study. This means that the treatment given in the trial may not be optimal.

This problematic design is linked to a wider challenge. The quality of the treatment/intervention is a central point in any CAM trial. In a research team housing a CAM practitioner and an academic researcher, it is often expected that the CAM practitioner will claim responsibility for the suitability of the intervention. However, there are sometimes obstacles to this arrangement. Usually the choice of design is heavily influenced or even governed by the academic researcher in view of their experience in planning studies. As a result, the design often involves a standardisation of the intervention leading to the loss of important aspects such as the number of medicines administered, the length of follow-up and restrictions in the handling of patients. It can be difficult for the CAM practitioner to object to this standardisation as it is frequently a prerequisite of the methodology.

In light of these difficulties, it is fair to suggest that the collaboration between CAM practitioner and academic researcher does not always form the basis of a good research team. Ideally, the role and level of input in decision-making of different parties will depend upon the power relations within the research team. As the experience of early CAM multidisciplinary practice models suggests, this is often an issue that despite best intentions can raise much concern and requires extensive attention if it is to be resolved (Budd et al. 1990, Paterson and Peacock 1995).

Conclusion

As this chapter has identified, a number of issues face both the individual CAM practitioner initiating research into their own therapy and the wider CAM community in their efforts to enhance the research capacity within practitioner ranks. CAM, like all areas of health care, is increasingly moving towards an evidence-based approach (Bondurant and Sox 2005), and this will bring rewards for CAM practitioners, at least in the eyes of the conventional medical community.

However, it is important that CAM practitioners do not become isolated from the developing research agenda and that their potential role within CAM research is acknowledged. CAM practitioners can provide the means for bridging the gap between practice and research, and their involvement in research can ensure the necessary capacity-building required to develop an appropriate multidisciplinary team approach to CAM investigation. Ultimately, the efforts of individual practitioners need to continue to be married with wide-ranging and systematic programmes and strategies for developing the research skills and experience of CAM practitioners. This will prove beneficial for not only CAM practitioners but all members of the CAM research community, irrespective of their background or disciplinary affiliations.

References

Adams, J. (2004) 'Demarcating the medical/non-medical border: occupational boundary-work within general practitioners' accounts of their integrative practice', in P. Tovey, G. Easthope and J. Adams (eds) *The Mainstreaming of Complementary and Alternative Medicine: Studies in Social Context*, London: Routledge, pp. 140–57.

Adams, J. and Tovey, P. (2000) 'Complementary medicine and primary care: towards a grassroots focus', in P. Tovey (ed.) *Contemporary Primary Care: The Challenge of Change*, Buckingham: Open University Press, pp. 167–82.

Andrews, G. T. (2004) 'Sharing the spirit of the policy agenda? Private complementary therapists' attitudes towards practising in the British NHS', *Complementary Therapies in Nursing and Midwifery*, 10 (4): 217–28.

—— (2006) 'Encouraging additional research capacity as an intellectual enterprise: extending Ernst's argument', *Complementary Therapies in Clinical Practice*, 12 (1): 13–17.

Angell, M. and Kassirer, J. P. (1998) 'Alternative medicine: the risks of untested and unregulated remedies', *New England Journal of Medicine*, 339 (12): 839–41.

Barnes, J., Abbot, N. C., Harkness, E. and Ernst, E. (1996) 'Articles on complementary medicine in the mainstream medical literature: an investigation of Medline, 1966 through 1996', *Archives of Internal Medicine*, 159 (15): 1721–5.

Barnes, P. M., Powell-Griner, E., McFann, K. and Nahin, R. L. (2004) 'Complementary and alternative medicine use among adults: United States, 2002', *Advances in Data*, 343 (3431): 1–19.

Bensoussan, A. and Lewith, G. T. (2004) 'Complementary medicine research in Australia: a strategy for the future', *Medical Journal of Australia*, 181 (6): 331–3.

Bondurant, S. and Sox, H. C. (2005) 'Mainstream and alternative medicine: converging paths require common standards', *Annals of Internal Medicine*, 142 (2): 149–50.

Botting, D. A. and Cook, R. (2000) 'Complementary medicine: knowledge, use and attitudes of doctors', *Complementary Therapies in Nursing and Midwifery*, 6 (1): 41–7.

Budd, C., Fischer, B., Parrinder, D. and Price, L. (1990) 'A model of co-operation between complementary and allopathic medicine in a primary care setting', *British Journal of General Practice*, 40 (338): 376–8.

Casey, M. G., Adams, J. and Sibbritt, D. (in press) 'An examination of the prescription and dispensing of medicines by Western herbal therapists: a national survey in Australia', *Complementary Therapies in Medicine*.

Coulter, I. D. and Willis, E. M. (2004) 'The rise and rise of complementary and alternative medicine: a sociological perspective', *Medical Journal of Australia*, 180 (11): 587–9.

Eisenberg, D. M., Davis, R. B., Ettner, S. L., Appel, S., Wilkey, S., Van Rompay, M. and Kessler, R. C. (1998) 'Trends in alternative medicine use in the United States, 1990–1997: results of a follow-up national survey', *Journal of the American Medical Association*, 280 (18): 1569–75.

Ernst, E. (2005) 'Keynote comment: dumbing down of complementary medicine', *Lancet Oncology*, 6 (7): 442–3.

Fonnebo, V. (2003) 'Forskning innen alternative medisin – ma vi finne opp nye metoder?', *Forskning*. Available online at <http://www.forskning.no/Artikler/2003/november/1068819412.14>.

Giannelli, M., Cuttini, M., Arniani, S., Baldi, P. and Buiatti, E. (2004) 'Le medicine non convenzionali in Toscana: attitudini e utilizzo nella popolazione [Alternative medicine in Toscana]', *Epidemiology and Prevention*, 28 (1): 27–33.

Goldstein, M. (2002) 'The emerging socioeconomic and political support for alternative medicine in the United States', *Annals of the American Academy of Political and Social Science*, 583 (1): 44–63.

Hanssen, B., Grimsgaard, S., Launso, L., Fonnebo, V., Falkenberg, T. and Rasmussen, N. K. R. (2005) 'Use of complementary and alternative medicine in Scandianavian countries', *Scandinavian Journal of Primary Health Care*, 23 (1): 57–62.

Harris, P. and Rees, R. (2000) 'The prevalence of complementary and alternative medicine use among the general population: a systematic review of the literature', *Complementary Therapies in Medicine*, 8 (2): 88–96.

Hsiao, A., Ryan, G. W., Hays, R. D., Coulter, I. D., Andersen, R. M. and Wenger, N. S. (2006) 'Variations in provider conceptions of integrative medicine', *Social Science and Medicine*, 62 (12): 2973–87.

Hunt, V., Randle, J. and Freshwater, D. (2004) 'Paediatric nurses' attitudes to massage and aromatherapy massage', *Complementary Therapies in Nursing and Midwifery*, 10 (3): 194–201.

Kinsel, J. F. and Straus, S. (2003) 'Complementary and alternative therapeutics: rigorous research is needed to support claims', *Annual Review of Pharmacology and Toxicology*, 43: 463–84.

Kotsirilos, V. (2005) 'Complementary and alternative medicine. Part 2: evidence and implications for GPs', *Australian Family Physician*, 34 (8): 689–91.

Leung, B., Verhoef, M. J. and Dryden, T. (2005) 'Mentoring programmes within a network to build research literacy and capacity in complementary and alternative medicine (CAM) practitioners', *Journal of Complementary and Integrative Medicine*, 2(1): article 9. (http://www.bepress.com/jcim/vol2/iss1/9).

Lewith, G. T. and Holgate, S. (2000) 'CAM research and development', *Complementary Therapies in Nursing and Midwifery*, 6 (1): 19–24.

Lewith, G. T., Jonas, W. B. and Walach, H. (2003) *Clinical Research in Complementary Therapies: Principles, Problems and Solutions*, Oxford: Churchill Livingstone.

Linde, K., Clausius, N., Ramirez, G., Melchart, D., Eitel, F., Hedges, L. V. and Jonas, W. B. (1997) 'Are the clinical effects of homoeopathy placebo effects? A meta-analysis of placebo-controlled trials', *Lancet*, 350 (9081): 834–43.

Lokken, P., Straumsheim, P. A., Tveiten, D., Skjelbred, P. and Borchgrevink, C. F. (1995) 'Effect of homoeopathy on pain and other events after acute trauma: placebo controlled trial with bilateral oral surgery', *British Medical Journal*, 310 (6992): 1439–42.

Mathie, R. T. (2003) 'The research evidence base for homoeopathy: a fresh assessment of the literature', *Homoeopathy*, 92 (2): 84–91.

McIvor, G. (1995) 'Practitioner research in probation', in J. McGuire (ed.) *What Works? Reducing Offending*, New York: Wiley.

McLeod, J. (1999) *Practitioner Research in Counselling*, London: Sage.

National Center for Complementary and Alternative Medicine (2004), 'CAM Practitioner Research Education Project Grant Partnership'. Available online at <http://grants.nih.gov/grants/pa-files/PAR–04–097.html>. (Accessed April 2006.)

Norges Offentlige Utredninger (1998) *Alternative Medisin, NOU 1998–2001 [Report on Alternative Medicine]*, Oslo: Statens Trykning, Statens Forvaltningstjenste.

Norske Homeopaters Landsforbund (1997) *Strategi for forskning pa homeopati [A Strategy for Research in Homoeopathy]*, Oslo: Norkse Homeopater Landsforbund.

Paterson, C. and Peacock, W. (1995) 'Complementary practitioners as part of the primary health care team: evaluation of one model', *British Journal of General Practice*, 45 (394): 255–8.

Raschetti, R., Menniti-Ippolito, F., Forcella, E. and Bianchi, C. (2005) 'Complementary and alternative medicine in the scientific literature', *Journal of Alternative and Complementary Medicine*, 11 (1): 209–12.

Steinsbekk, A. and Fonnebo, V. (2003) 'Users of homoeopathy in Norway in 1998 compared to previous users and GP patients', *Homoeopathy*, 92 (1): 3–10.

Straumsheim, P. (1990) 'Homeopatisk behanlding av 20 pasienter med recidiverende Nedre Urinveisinfeksjon (NUI) [Homeopathic treatment of twenty patients with recurrent lower urinary tract infection]', *Dynamis*, 1: 8–9.

Tiran, D. (2006) 'Complementary therapies in pregnancy: midwives' and obstetricians' appreciation of risk', *Complementary Therapies in Clinical Practice*, 12 (2): 126–31.

Tovey, P., Easthope, G. and Adams, J. (eds) (2004) *The Mainstreaming of Complementary and Alternative Medicine: Studies in Social Context*, London: Routledge.

Wilder, B. and Ernst, E. (2003) 'CAM research funding in the UK: surveys of medical charities in 1999 and 2002', *Complementary Therapies in Medicine*, 11 (3): 165–7.

Zick, M. and Benn, R. (2004) 'Bridging CAM practice and research: teaching CAM practitioners about research methodology', *Alternative Therapies in Health and Medicine*, 10 (3): 50–6.

Chapter 8

Public health and CAM

Exploring overlap, contrast
and dissonance

Kevin Dew and Penelope Carroll

Introduction

From a public-health perspective, there are a number of important issues raised by CAM. As with clinical medicine, CAM and public health do not and will not necessarily have an easy or friction-free relationship. There is a great deal of research and commentary on particular aspects of CAM and public health, especially in relation to issues of efficacy, regulation, access and use of CAM practices.[1] Bodeker and Kronenberg (2002) suggest that these issues need to be seen within a broader social, cultural and economic context and that the public-health dimensions of CAM need to be defined. This chapter attempts to contribute to this debate by focusing on different frameworks used by public health and CAM for understanding health and disease. This is to promote understanding of the disparate perspectives and to suggest some ways in which CAM perspectives are significant for public health.

There are some obvious reasons why CAM and public health come into conflict. Public health tends to develop standardised or uniform solutions for whole populations, therefore it is difficult to accommodate difference and diversity. In many instances, CAM takes a unique approach to each individual. In this light, the kind of answers to health problems that CAM and public health produce can be contrasting, and at times in opposition. We can think of many examples, such as the issue of pasteurisation of milk and cheese, fluoridation of water and universal vaccinations. In these examples, public health has pushed for the universal treatment of a food, the universal addition of a substance to an essential commodity and the universal application of a treatment to healthy people. From different CAM perspectives, these universal measures can be problematic.

For pasteurisation, some claim that the process of 'boiling up milk' means many nutrients are lost (Jeffreys 1998: 253). With fluoridation, some claim that it causes disease such as osteosarcoma and that its protective properties are overstated (see Martin 1991 for an in-depth discussion of the fluoridation controversy). Members of different CAM professions have at times seen the protective properties of vaccines as overstated and have regarded vaccination as a toxic attack on the body, lowering the responsiveness of the immune system (Chaitow 1987).

Coulter (2004) suggests that the concept of naturalism is associated with many CAM groups. Coulter argues that 'there is a widespread acceptance of things natural' (2004: 113), and, for some, being closer to that natural state is better. From a public-health perspective, being closer to a natural state may increase the risk of infections or provide insufficient amounts of some vital or important element (see Petersen and Lupton 1996 for a discussion of discourses on nature and risk). There is, however, another public-health perspective that has developed in response to attempts to understand the increase in asthma and other allergic conditions in the Western world. This has become known as the hygiene hypothesis, which suggests that infections during infancy protect against these conditions, and that the use of antibiotics and paracetamol may increase the risk of asthma (Cohet et al. 2004). As such, the efforts to shield people from 'nature' are seen as having some negative consequences.

We can see quite distinctively different representations of nature in this debate, where nature can be viewed as either benign or dangerous. The status of 'natural' changes too. The boundaries between nature and culture can be somewhat indistinct, and things that are seen as 'natural' in one time or place can be seen as medical conditions at another (White 1999).

Another distinctive difference between CAM and public health is around the goal of interventions. For public health, the goal is quite simply measurable population declines in the level of morbidity and mortality (and when combined with health economics, the goal is how to do this in the most resource-efficient manner). As such, there is no clear notion of what health is within public health (in its epidemiologic manifestations). With CAM, interventions may aim at allowing patients to achieve 'their full potential in light of their biological, psycho-social and spiritual limitations' (Coulter 2004: 114). This extends the 1957 World Health Organisation (WHO) definition of health as 'a condition or quality of the human organism which expresses adequate functioning under given genetic and environmental conditions' (cited in Grbich 1999: 7). There may also be a dimension in CAM that 'relates the human being to its past and future, it emphasizes the goal-striving behaviour, the realization of the self over time' (Aakster 1986: 268). Related to different notions of health are different notions of disease. In a biomedical model, disease is perceived as a physical malfunction that must be corrected or an infestation that must be removed. Sickness is not something that happens to 'whole human beings but something that happens to their parts' (White 1999: 36). Other models may see disease as the outcome of biological, psychological and social processes, or even spiritual influences (Dew 2001).

Exploring case studies: perspectives from the field

To further illustrate the potential tensions between CAM perspectives and public health, three examples will be explored in more depth: the case of immunisation, the place of indigenous healing practices and, finally, alternative conceptions of public health. While these three areas do not always necessarily draw directly upon exploring CAM practice and consumption, they have been chosen to help illuminate a number of positions and perspectives that often accompany or overlap CAM perspectives.

Rather than just note potential challenges, the discussion will also highlight the productive nature of these tensions in relation to public health and CAM research agendas. These examples are all taken from our ongoing work and, as such, are all located in New Zealand. However, the general arguments are also applicable to public health and CAM in other countries.

Immunisation and its resistance

The practice of vaccination to confer immunity or protection from infectious disease is held in such high regard that it is presented as a cornerstone of preventative medicine (Streefland 2001). The first widely used vaccine was that commonly considered to have eradicated small pox worldwide. Today there are a variety of vaccines, many of which are incorporated into vaccination programmes for children. In some jurisdictions these are mandatory, while in others they are supported by strong coercive campaigns to increase the uptake of vaccination (Dew 1999). New vaccines are added to the schedule on a regular basis, so in addition to the core vaccines for mumps, measles, rubella, diphtheria, poliomyelitis and tetanus, over the past decade new ones for varicella, haemophilus influenzae type B and meningococcal meningitis may also be included.

From a public-health perspective, vaccinations are a good use of resources, based on calculations relating the costs of the intervention to the perceived benefits conferred. Those supporting the introduction of new vaccines, such as the meningococcal meningitis vaccine recently introduced into New Zealand, have to convince the public and politicians of their value, and arguments put forward by policy-makers can be, and are, contested (for examples of the contested nature of the debate see the Immunisation Awareness Society web site <http://www.ias.org.nz>). For the use of routine vaccines, research issues from a public-health perspective focus on how to increase vaccine coverage. This research can include obtaining the rationales of those who do and do not vaccinate their children. From a public-health perspective, the latter may be seen as having an irrational response. However, in the social-science research in this area, the interpretation of responses is somewhat different. For example, Rogers and Pilgrim (1995) argue that representations of vaccinations and disease vary according to the social location of different groups, with health promotion groups and dissenting parents taking diametrically opposed views. Similarly, Streefland (2001) argues that non-acceptors may have sound reasons for their stand and have the same concerns about protecting the health of their children as acceptors.

A very powerful concept that promotes efforts to obtain universal, or near universal, population coverage of vaccines is that of herd immunity (Tobias et al. 1987). Greater benefits can be conferred, even on those who are not vaccinated, if herd immunity is achieved. In addition, it is believed that if herd immunity is achieved, particular diseases can be completely eradicated.

It is not surprising, therefore, that due to the sanctity conferred on vaccinations, there is a relatively small number of conscientious objectors. Although it is estimated that in New Zealand only 60 per cent of children complete the vaccination schedule, it is thought that less than 6 per cent of those are unvaccinated as a result of a conscious choice (Hamilton et al. 2004). What may be of concern from a public-health perspective is that the increasing popularity of CAM could result in an increase in those objecting to vaccines. Historically, the medical profession has strongly attacked CAM groups because of their stance on vaccines (Dew 2003).

So where could public-health researchers interested in CAM go with this apparent gulf between the two perspectives? There are a number of possibilities. Instead of dismissing claims by some CAM groups or individuals as irrational, the methodologies of public health could be used to explore the claims in more depth. For example, can we see different patterns of disease and health-service utilisation in people who have chosen not to vaccinate? This may prove difficult as we would need to control for differences in socioeconomic status, ethnicity, gender, education and perhaps other factors. The tools of epidemiology – pitched very much at the concerns of public health to reduce morbidity and mortality – may be able to answer that question to some extent, although it would be no easy task. The social-science skills within public health could also be used to explore concerns about adverse vaccination events. Qualitative data could be collected from those who claim adverse effects to explore not only the claims made, but also the responses of medical professionals and the compensation/insurance systems to those claims. Some limited quantitative data is available,[2] but in New Zealand this relies on voluntary reporting of adverse reactions by GPs and therefore may not be particularly reliable. Such information may provide a better picture of the extent or understanding of adverse events and may generate further hypotheses about the vaccination issue that could be tested. This information could then feed back into the assessment of costs and benefits of vaccines.

From a public-health policy perspective, there is a range of options for research, including the exploration of the influences on decisions to develop and incorporate new vaccines into immunisation schedules. The recent campaign to develop a meningococcal meningitis vaccine in New Zealand would make an interesting case study in this regard – particularly given the very different representations of the issue that have surfaced. Another research strategy here would be to explore the role and experiences of dissenting scientists. The case of autism and the measles–mumps–rubella vaccine (MMR) in the UK would be a useful example here. Finally, any claims for protection against disease conferred by CAM interventions could be assessed, either using the standard EBM measures or developing new methodologies in collaboration with CAM practitioners making such claims.

There are opportunities for public health and CAM researchers to provide a bridge between sometimes very hostile camps by using research skills to explore the fascinating and emotionally charged topic of vaccinations in more depth.

Indigenous healing practices

When CAM practices are discussed it is not common to include the health and healing practices of indigenous populations in settler societies (for example, New Zealand, Australia and Canada) or the particular health practices of immigrant groups to Western countries. Nevertheless, such practices can be identified as sharing some core similarities to CAM, especially in terms of their traditional political exclusion from mainstream health organisation. In this section, the term 'indigenous' is used to describe first nations peoples, that is, people who live in a country that has been colonised. We could extend the term 'indigenous practices' to include the use of folk remedies by European peoples or people of European descent, and while some of these practices form the basis of current CAM practices (Hand 1980) they are not the focus of this chapter.

In terms of health-services delivery, the position of indigenous healing practices can be a significant issue, particularly if a society is committed (whether rhetorically or in reality) to acknowledging the value of the indigenous culture. The relationship between indigenous health practices and mainstream medicine can be illustrated in interesting ways by exploring the example of New Zealand.

In New Zealand, the Treaty of Waitangi (signed in 1840 and regarded as the founding document of the nation) plays an important role in the position of healing practices. The treaty was signed by representatives of the British crown and Maori iwi (or tribes) and gave Maori the same citizenship rights as other British subjects. The treaty contains three clauses that guarantee Maori certain rights in relation to the crown. The first clause relates to the crown's responsibilities in relation to governance; the second clause relates to Maori autonomy and self-determination; and the third clause guarantees Maori the same rights as non-Maori citizens (Signal et al. 2004).

From a public-health perspective, a major focus in relation to indigenous health has been the disparity in health outcomes between Maori and non-Maori in New Zealand, where for almost all health outcomes Maori are worse off in terms of morbidity and mortality (Salmond and Crampton 2000, Ajwani et al. 2003). The gap in health outcomes has led to much work exploring the reasons for such a gap, focusing on various social determinants of health, including socio-economic differences, racism and the history of colonialism (Dew and Kirkman 2002, Ajwani et al. 2003).

In Australia, too, research in Aboriginal health shows Aboriginal people have consistently higher health risks, disability, morbidity and mortality across all age groups relative to non-Aboriginal people, with a life expectancy fifteen to twenty years lower (Anderson 1999). From the time of the first Aboriginal health service set up in Redfern, Sydney, in 1972, Aboriginal community-controlled health services have embedded principles of self-determination and 'creat[ing] an Aboriginal space within the health system' (Anderson 1999: 67).

There has also been the development of many Maori health providers as a response to this issue of gaps in health outcomes and to the broader issue of honouring the Treaty of Waitangi in providing services that respect Maori autonomy and self-determination. Within mainstream institutions, particular cultural services have been provided since the early 1980s in mental-health services. These have included aspects of traditional healing such as the use of *karakia* (prayer) and *mirimiri* (massage) (Cunningham and Durie 2005). There has been an understanding that the European therapeutic goal of an independent, self-actualised individual does not necessarily fit the Maori paradigm. From the 1970s, Maori had begun to insist that a narrow bio-medical focus was not a good foundation for health delivery or planning and emphasised the value of traditional beliefs, but not necessarily at the expense of Western medical practice. What gained acceptance as 'the Maori health perspective' was a health construct incorporating the spiritual (*taha wairua*), mental (*taha hinengaro*) and physical (*taha tinana*), along with extended family (*taha whanau*). This was a construct that acknowledged the importance of tribal landownership (*mana whenua*) to Maori health and well-being (Durie 1999). Biomedical models also provide only a partial account of health and well-being from an Aboriginal perspective, with the concept of *punya* encompassing physical, cultural, social, emotional and spiritual elements of the individual, the wider community and the land (Anderson 1999). An explanation of health and well-being which links the individual with social and supernatural environments, as both Maori and Aboriginal health concepts do, 'is still the most commonly held explanation of the cause of illness worldwide' (Grbich 1999: 8).

With the biomedical model dominating New Zealand and Australian health delivery, there is clearly a conflict with traditional indigenous views of health and well-being. From a public-health perspective, research questions in relation to these developments in Maori health-service provision and the use of traditional methods of healing would relate to the way in which they may lead to improvements in health. Getting a measure of this is notoriously difficult, and broader notions of health than the traditional objective measures collected by epidemiologists would need to be considered.

However, the existence of traditional healing practices alongside biomedical practices does provide an opportunity for other avenues of research. For example, how are these services used? How are choices made as to which approach is appropriate? And are the different approaches able to be integrated or are they kept separate? There has been little published research in this area.

At a broader level still, are indigenous practices conferred a legitimacy in the health system? If so, does this provide an avenue for greater conferral of legitimacy to other CAM practices? It should be noted here that orthodox health practitioners might also confer legitimacy on CAM when they use CAM procedures in the diagnosis and treatment of disease. There are many general practitioners who use CAM (Dew 2003) along with other health professionals such as nurses and physiotherapists.

In terms of research processes and specifically methodological issues, there is much that can be gained from the consideration of indigenous peoples' understandings and practices. At one level there are critiques from indigenous academics of the epistemological foundations of Western research. Walker (2004) argues that the nature of the scientific community and its attitudes to indigenous knowledge disadvantage Maori knowledge and that 'indigenous peoples internationally have had to struggle for acknowledgement of their knowledge base' (Walker 2004: 112). Anderson (1999) shows how this has been the case in Australia, with knowledge about Aboriginal people stemming in part from cultural traditions in early colonial times which meant that: 'whereas settlers saw themselves as civilised, industrious and individualised, Aborigines were seen to be primitive, lazy and over social or tribal.' He highlights persistent themes in the 'colonial metaphor for Aboriginality [as] . . . a somewhat pathetic and bewildered primitive people trapped by the advance of western civilisation' (Anderson 1999: 56).

A more ontological aspect to this field of inquiry is the way in which 'secular' scientists separate the spiritual world from the natural world. One Maori participant in a study of informal housing and health (Carroll forthcoming) talked of 'spiritual DNA': '[The land] is where we come from, this is our mother, so we have a spiritual connection. That's what *mauri* is. Everything's got *mauri*, animate and inanimate . . . what it is basically is spiritual DNA' (Carroll forthcoming). A further facet is the relationship between collective and individual knowledge, ancestral knowledge and present-day knowledge. The difference between the *iwi* (tribal) way of knowing and scientific knowledge is highlighted: 'There's tacit knowledge and explicit knowledge. Explicit knowledge is something you know because you've been taught it; tacit knowledge is something you just know' (Carroll forthcoming). Walker states 'Maori don't choose to hold on to the values of the ancestors, the values of the ancestors hold on to us if we are lucky enough to hear them in the many songs, pepeha, haka and other oral literature' (Walker 2004: 215). As such, oral tradition is a source of knowledge in a way that is not the case for the objectifying science that informs much of public-health research.

In addition, 'Papatuanuku [the earth mother] is a living thing: it is not separate from the individual and the individual is not separate from the collective' (Walker 2004: 215). The holistic view expressed here provides some major challenges for public-health research. Researchers are not only dealing with mechanisms of causation that might be different from orthodox ones but are dealing with completely different epistemologies and ontologies. Public-health researchers need to consider this fundamental issue when wanting to research issues related to indigenous understandings and health practices and would need to work alongside experienced indigenous researchers who are steeped in the two worlds (indigenous and Western) in order to better appreciate the complex relationships between health, well-being, disease and worldviews.

These different epistemological and ontological perspectives have real consequences for data collection in public-health research. For instance, the SF36 health-status questionnaire, used widely internationally as a self-report measure of health, has a two-dimensional structure with distinct mental and physical health components. A study by Scott et al. (2000) evaluated the possibility that this separation of the mental and physical would not be supported by Maori and Pacific ethnic groups in New Zealand, whose models of health are more holistic. Their analysis showed that this was the case and that for Pacific peoples and Maori forty-five years and over the physical and mental health components were not clearly differentiated by the two-dimensional structure of the questionnaire (Scott et al. 2000).

These differences in epistemological and ontological perspectives are a rich source of material for research but they also alert us to the need to thoroughly interrogate the data-collection tools we use to ensure that we capture the variety of ways of experiencing and understanding health and well-being.

Alternative public health

A challenge to what could be called orthodox public-health positions can come from a variety of other views that provide a different perspective on health. Some of these views are aligned with CAM concepts, such as ideas of naturalism and holism. In an attempt to illustrate the variety of perspectives, five positions are discussed in this section. It is not claimed here that these positions are exhaustive of all views on health or that they are mutually exclusive. For any particular individual, they could well overlap and people could change positions depending on circumstances. To add further complexity, it may be appropriate to see these positions as not either/or, but as constituting a continuum, where people may have more or less of one 'position' than another. What follows is a brief characterisation of the five positions with an illustration of how each one could relate to the issue of immunisation.

Utilitarian

This is the 'orthodox' public-health position whereby the concern is to increase longevity and decrease morbidity. From a population-health perspective this may mean on occasions accepting that some individuals may suffer, but that this is for the greater good, and that overall the quantum of health benefits will outweigh the quantum of suffering. This might characterise someone who chooses to immunise or not immunise based on the contribution this will make to the community or population health.

Risk averse

This position shares similar concerns to the utilitarian position, but in this case the focus is on the individual avoiding risks and suffering and not on overall population health gains. This might characterise someone who chooses to immunise or not immunise on the grounds of personal risks.

Realistic hedonism

This is where health is not conceptualised as the avoidance of disease and where longevity in itself is not a goal. The goal is to live life to the full, accepting that there is always a downside – to experience the world, to embrace suffering as one strand in the rich tapestry of human existence. The issue of immunisation is unlikely to have any clear relationship to this position.

Purist

This is where there may be similar concerns about longevity to those characterising realistic hedonism, but in this case the focus is on what is wholesome and pure. Contamination of the body is avoided, which includes the ingestion of toxic drugs. Immunisation may be avoided due to a view that it introduces a toxic element to the body. From this perspective, the body would be supported in a 'natural' way to fight off diseases.

Holism

This is where one's individual health is only seen in relation to a broader dimension of environmental health. One's actions then should enhance the environment and not cause damage. Both environmentalists and indigenous health beliefs espouse this view. The focus on the environment may be related to protecting individuals but is seen within the context of ecosystems. The issue of immunisation may be quite complex in this position and it is possible that using vaccines may be seen as disrupting evolutionary principles or damaging the balance of life on earth.

As stated, these are not exhaustive of all possible positions in relation to personal and public health. For example, others may incorporate different forms of fatalism, notions of God's will and karmic influences. Also, as stated, these are not exclusive; one can be utilitarian and risk averse, or utilitarian and purist. But at times these positions can be in opposition and, in particular, the population-health perspective of the utilitarian model could clash with the realistic hedonism, holistic and purist perspectives. This can be illustrated with research currently being undertaken in New Zealand on housing and health (Howden-Chapman and Crane 2004).

As part of this wider research programme, interviews were conducted with people who were in informal housing. Informal housing includes staying in garages, caravans and tents, old buses, house trucks and sheds and sleeping rough. Those in the study living in informal housing in a rural area have made a positive choice to return to the land. They have rejected the comforts of urban life and live in accommodation that is sub-standard from a public-health perspective. That is, they may have no running water in their dwelling, no mains electricity, no insulation, no sewerage system. Instead they may be using long-drop toilets, collect their water from a nearby stream or spring or use rainwater off the roof), make do with candles and battery-powered lighting and heat water and cook on wood-fired stoves or with bottled gas. Many promote a rhetoric of hardiness, where city living makes people soft and where people have no real experience of living. These informants claim that living back on the land hardens you, makes you more resilient and enhances your experience of life. What others may see as suffering can be rearticulated as part of the process of toughening up and gaining access to the experience of living life to the full.

There is also a strong spiritual aspect. Maori and Pakeha alike speak of the health-giving connection with nature and beauty, their interconnectedness with the bush, the land, streams and the sea. Living on the land and from the land and sea (in terms of growing food, fishing and collecting shellfish) and caring for the land, are seen as health-promoting and essential for their well-being. Maori, in addition, articulate a sense of oneness with the land of their ancestors, their childhood and their present-day *whanau* (family) and *turangawaewae* (place to stand). There is also a strong environmental awareness with some, a rejection of the mainstream materialist values which are identified as leading to a plundering of natural resources and widespread pollution. The emphasis is on conservation, regeneration and using as few resources as possible. Realistic hedonism and holistic perspectives combine in these people living in informal housing.

By contrast, research is also being undertaken to develop a healthy housing index. Since the nineteenth century, housing conditions and public health have been inextricably linked, with a correlation between poor housing and poor health. From this perspective, informal accommodation with sub-standard services will be identified as poor housing that people should not live in, and that someone should have the responsibility for ensuring that all people live in adequate housing, as determined by the index. Research has shown links between damp, cold, mouldy houses and respiratory illness, and a retrofit programme carried out by the Housing and Health Research pro-gramme (Howden-Chapman et al. in press) demonstrates the direct health improvements resulting from houses being insulated. The clash between the latter's utilitarian view and the more realistic hedonism/holistic views of the former is obvious. None of the participants in the informal housing study are living in dwellings that comply with building and health and safety regula-tions. None of them is living in a permitted dwelling. Does this mean they are putting themselves or others at risk?

From a mainstream public-health perspective, personal and public health risks of informal housing are readily identified. These include:

- risks from the unsafe use of gas bottles, candles and open fires;
- injury risks from living in structurally unsound dwellings;
- health risks from living in uninsulated, cold and damp dwellings;
- personal and environmental risks resulting from a lack of reticulated water and the use of alternative toilet facilities;
- and environmental problems caused by grey water discharge (discharge from baths and showers, from washing dishes, floors, clothes and so on).

Those living in informal housing have their own perspectives on and responses to health risks. This includes identifying ways to minimise the danger from open fires and candles; a view that their dwellings are not unsafe and that they are warmer and less damp than many conventional houses; that composting toilets and properly maintaining long drops are good ecological options that help conserve water and a presentation of strong environmental ethics in relation to grey-water discharges.

Public-health measures such as fluoridated and chlorinated water supplies, reticulated sewage systems and septic tanks and mains electricity were rejected by these individuals, although there was recognition that such measures could be necessary in an urban environment because of population density. For them, in their informal housing situations, these were seen variously as unnecessary, wasteful of resources, polluting and expensive. Light and noise 'pollution' were seen as additional drawbacks to mainstream living. The pref-erence for spring-, stream- or rainwater rather than treated town-supply water was universal.

In addition, those living in informal housing found the financial pressures of mortgages and rents unhealthy and would emphasise the health benefits of

their situations. They highlighted the health-enhancing beauty of their sur-
roundings, interconnectedness with the land and living in harmony with
nature.

This study raises questions about mainstream public health: Do we need to
broaden our views about what is health-promoting? Do we need to take into
account more of the realistic hedonism and holistic perspectives in research
and not focus so narrowly on utilitarian views? With particular regard
to informal housing, can public-health researchers inform policy-makers
about the implications of taking a 'one size fits all' ethos, for example in
relation to building regulations?[3] In addition, an awareness of the very different perspectives that people take about public and personal health can be a
fruitful research topic in its own right. The challenge here is to deepen our
understanding of alternative public-health positions (including those around
CAM), perhaps to consider how different views may be patterned in the
population and to consider the implications of these diverse perspectives
in relation to receptivity to public-health interventions. For public-health
researchers, an awareness of alternative public-health perspectives may lead
to a reconsideration of universal measures to overcome identified health
problems.

Research issues arising

There are many interesting issues that come out of exploring the research
relationships between CAM and public health. Some of the issues are
cautionary. Public-health researchers need to be cautious about applying
standard measures of health. People from a variety of perspectives may
assess health in different ways. In this chapter we have discussed indigenous
perspectives and alternative public-health perspectives. This suggests that the
development of more sophisticated data-collection tools for public health
that can take into account and give voice to these different perspectives is
important.

Second, CAM and public-health researchers could work to deepen our
understanding of these different perspectives and their implications for health-
seeking and sustaining behaviours. This suggests the need for multidisciplinary research to try to enhance the chances of researchers from different
disciplines gaining a greater insight into the concepts used and the perspectives
taken in relation to health, measurement and understanding.

Third, we need a greater understanding of the underlying values of public
health. This chapter has suggested that an orthodox public-health perspective
is utilitarian, with the values of universalism lying at its foundation. There is
little exploration of the concept of health and a narrow focus in terms of
measurement. But there is much more that could be explored in relation
to the underlying values of public health, such as the concept of risk and
the classification systems deployed. In addition, social-research strategies

could be used to shed greater light on the politics of public health, to better understand why particular issues gain traction in public-health research consciousness and, perhaps, why CAM and related perspectives on the whole have not.

Fourth, this chapter suggests that it is fruitful to explore the ways in which different perspectives, such as CAM and public health, can be accommodated. Can researchers provide a bridge between the different camps in the vaccination debate? How can we combine indigenous and other health perspectives, the individual and the universal, different views in relation to sanitation and housing? Will the development of such things as a healthy housing index result in increased attack and opposition to alternative views of living? And if so, what are the implications for health and well-being?

Finally, public-health researchers, particularly those with a health-services focus, could explore in depth how health professionals accommodate different perspectives, such as EBM, CAM, patient-centred and indigenous perspectives. This can apply to how health professionals work with these perspectives in their own practice and also how they respond to patients who emphasise a perspective that may not easily align with their own. Exploring such research issues would lend itself to in-depth observation studies of social interaction in order to understand how health professionals respond in practice to the presentation of different perspectives. Analysis of such interactions could also explore whether and how people simultaneously hold contradictory views around personal and public health.

We can also note similarities in some of the assumptions of public health and both indigenous and alternative public-health perspectives that are in some sense oppositional to both CAM and biomedical practices. In social epidemiology there is an interest in how aspects of social organisation (such as levels of inequality, discrimination, etc.) get 'under the skin', given the accepted view that these aspects of social organisation have an impact on health (Howden-Chapman 2005). As such, social epidemiology looks at a number of causal mechanisms. Some of these are described under the rubric of psycho-social causes (Brunner and Marmot 1999). To illustrate in what is perhaps an oversimplified fashion, being at the bottom of a hierarchy causes stress, and stress can have detrimental physiological effects that may increase the chances of becoming chronically ill or even lower resistance to infectious agents. Like public health, indigenous and some alternative health approaches also stress social and environmental impacts on health. This tends not to be the case with either biomedicine or CAM. Biomedicine focuses on drug-based treatments to deal with the symptoms, but leaves the distal social causes of the disease untouched. CAM provides a critique of biomedicine on these grounds (Coulter 2004: 112). However, while CAM does focus on causality, it tends to be in terms of such things as an individual's decline in vitality, a misalignment of the spine or a build-up of toxins in the body, rather than social conditions. As with biomedicine, intervention is based on individualised treatment and not efforts to address social issues. The discussion of indigenous and alternative public-health perspectives presented in this chapter suggests these may in many ways actually be closer to the social aspects of orthodox public health than both biomedicine and individualised CAM approaches. Certainly, the central role of the land or environment in health and well-being may readily overlap with public-health concerns about distal causes.

For CAM researchers, a consideration of the public-health dimensions of CAM may open up new audiences for their work. Public health, as an academic discipline, is founded on epidemiological research methods; CAM research using other approaches to knowledge generation, such as ethnographic research, can better inform epidemiologists so that their research design can take into consideration the broader social and cultural perspective of the use and experience of CAM. Greater interaction between CAM and public-health research could be of mutual benefit. Exploring overlaps, contrasts and dissonances between different health perspectives, such as orthodox public health and CAM, opens up a whole range of research strategies that have the potential to deepen our understanding of these quite different disciplines and their impact on health and well-being.

Acknowledgements

We would like to thank Dr Monika Clark-Grill and Professor Alistair Woodward for their insights on some of the issues raised in this chapter.

Notes

1 For example, a special edition of the *American Journal of Public Health* (2002, 92 [10]) is devoted to CAM and the health of the public; many articles also appear in such journals as *Complementary Therapies in Medicine* and the *Journal of Complementary and Alternative Medicine*.
2 In New Zealand the agency responsible for collating reported data on adverse reactions is the Centre for Adverse Reactions Monitoring. The web site for this agency is <http://www.otago.ac.nz/carm>. The web site states that 'it is estimated that only 5 per cent of all reactions are reported'.
3 From within a utilitarian public-health perspective there is also a potential clash with the introduction of more stringent standards in building codes. Protecting health and safety is the main rationale for having residential building codes, yet Hammitt et al. (1999) demonstrate that unintended health and safety risks may result when new regulations increase building costs: more expensive homes because of increased code-related costs can produce an 'income effect', drawing household income away from other health-protecting expenditure, and this can also produce a 'stock effect', with more people remaining in older, less healthy homes and putting off needed renovations because they cannot meet increased code-related costs.

References

Aakster, C. W. (1986) 'Concepts in alternative medicine', *Social Science and Medicine*, 22 (2): 265–73.

Ajwani, S., Blakely, T., Robson, R., Tobias, M. and Bonne, M. (2003) *Decades of Disparity: Ethnic Mortality Trends in New Zealand 1980–1999*, Wellington: Ministry of Health and the University of Otago.

Anderson, I. (1999) 'Aboriginal well-being', in C. Grbich (ed.) *Health in Australia: Sociological Concepts and Issues*, Sydney: Longman.

Bodeker, G. and Kronenberg, F. (2002) 'A public health agenda for traditional, complementary and alternative medicine', *American Journal of Public Health*, 92 (10): 1582–91.

Brunner, E. and Marmot, M. (1999) 'Social organization, stress and health', in M. Marmot and R. Wilkinson (eds) *Social Determinants of Health*, Oxford: Oxford University Press.

Chaitow, L. (1987) *Vaccination and Imminization: Dangers, Delusions and Alternatives*, Saffron Walden: C. W. Daniel.

Cohet, C., Cheng, S., MacDonald, C., Baker, M., Foliaki, S., Huntingdon, N., Douwes, J. and Pearce, N. (2004) 'Infections, medication use, and the prevalence of symptoms of asthma, rhinitis and eczema in childhood', *Journal of Epidemiology and Community Health*, 58 (10): 852–7.

Coulter, I. (2004) 'Integration and paradigm clash: the practical difficulties of integrative medicine', in P. Tovey, G. Easthope and J. Adams (eds) *The Mainstreaming of Complementary and Alternative Medicine: Studies in Social Context*, London: Routledge, 103–22.

Cunningham, C. and Durie, D. (2005) 'Te rerenga hauora', in K. Dew and P. Davis (eds) *Health and Society in Aotearoa/New Zealand*, Auckland: Oxford University Press.

Dew, K. (1999) 'Epidemics, panic and power: representations of measles and measles vaccines', *Health: An Interdisciplinary Journal for the Study of Health, Illness and Medicine*, 3 (4): 379–98.

—— (2001) 'Modes of practice and models of science in medicine', *Health: An Interdisciplinary Journal for the Study of Health, Illness and Medicine*, 5 (1): 93–111.

—— (2003) *Borderland Practices: Regulating Alternative Therapies in New Zealand*, Dunedin: University of Otago Press.

Dew, K. and Kirkman, A. (2002) *Sociology of Health in New Zealand*, Auckland: Oxford University Press.

Durie, M. (1999) *Whaiora*, Auckland: Oxford University Press.

Grbich, C. (1999) 'Approaches to health', in C. Grbich (ed). *Health in Australia: Sociological Concepts and Issues*, Sydney: Longman, pp. 4–9.

Hamilton, M., Corwin, P., Gower, S. and Rogers, S. (2004) 'Why do parents choose not to immunise their children', *New Zealand Medical Journal*, 117 (1189): 768.

Hammitt, K., Belsky, E., Levy, J. and Graham, J. (1999) 'Residential building codes, affordability, and health protection: a risk-trade off approach', *Risk Analysis*, 19 (6): 1037–58.

Hand, W. (1980) *Magical Medicine: The Folkloric Component of Medicine in the Folk*

Belief, Custom, and Ritual of the Peoples of Europe and America, Berkeley, Calif.: University of California Press.

Howden-Chapman, P. (2005) 'Unequal socio-economic determinants, unequal health', in K. Dew and P. Davis (eds) *Health and Society in Aotearoa New Zealand*, Melbourne: Oxford University Press.

Howden-Chapman, P. and Crane, J. (2004) 'Reducing health inequality through improving housing: He Kainga Oranga/ Housing and Health Research Programme', in P. Howden-Chapman and P. Carroll (eds) *Housing and Health: Research, Policy and Innovation*, Wellington: Steele Roberts.

Howden-Chapman, P., Crane, J., Matheson, A., Viggers, H., Cunningham, M., Blakely, T., O'Dea, D., Cunningham, C., Woodward, A., Saville-Smith, K., Baker, M. and Waipara, N. (2005) 'Retrofitting homes with insulation to reduce health inequalities: a clustered, randomised trial in community settings', *Social Science and Medicine*, 61 (12): 2600–10

Jeffreys, T. (1998) *Your Health at Risk: What Doctors and the Government Aren't Telling You*, Auckland: Howling at the Moon Publishing.

Martin, B. (1991) *Scientific Knowledge in Controversy: The Social Dynamics of the Fluoridation Debate*, Albany, NY: State University of New York Press.

Penelope, C. (forthcoming) 'Capturing Realities of Informal Housing', Ph.D. thesis, University of Victoria, Wellington.

Petersen, A. and Lupton, D. (1996) *The New Public Health: Health and Self in the Age of Risk*, St Leonards, NSW: Allen and Unwin.

Rogers, A. and Pilgrim, D. (1995) 'This risk of resistance: perspectives on the mass childhood immunisation programmes', in J. Gabe (ed.) *Medicine, Health and Risk: Sociological Approaches*, Oxford: Basil Blackwell, pp. 73–90.

Salmond, C. and Crampton, P. (2000) 'Deprivation in health', in P. Howden-Chapman and M. Tobias (eds) *Social Inequalities in Health: New Zealand 1999*, Wellington: Ministry of Health, pp. 9–63.

Scott, K., Sarfati, D., Tobias, M. and Haslett, S. (2000) 'A challenge to the cross-cultural validity of the SF-36 health survey: factor structure in Maori, Pacific and New Zealand European ethnic groups', *Social Science and Medicine*, 51 (11): 1655–64.

Signal, L., Rochford, T., Martin, J., Dew, K., Grant, M. and Howden-Chapman, P. (2004) 'Strengthening the capacity of mainstream organisations to tackle inequalities in health for Maori: a heart health case study', *Health Promotion Journal of Australia*, 15 (3): 221–5.

Streefland, P. (2001) 'Public doubts about vaccination safety and resistance against vaccination', *Health Policy*, 55 (3): 159–72.

Tobias, M., Scadden, J., Clements, J. and Patel, A. (1987) 'Measles immunity in children: the 1985 national immunisation survey', *New Zealand Medical Journal*, 100: 315–17.

Walker, T. (2004) 'Valuing Maori ways of knowing and being', in K. Dew and R. Fitzgerald (eds) *Challenging Science: Issues for New Zealand Society in the 21st Century*, Palmerston North: Dunmore Press.

White, K. (1999) 'The social origins of illness and the development of the sociology of health', in C. Grbich (ed.) *Health in Australia: Sociological Concepts and Issues*, Sydney: Longman.

Chapter 9

Involving the consumer in CAM research

Charlotte Paterson

Introduction

Consumer involvement helps to ensure that research focuses on issues important to patients and that research is conducted *with* patients and not *on* them. The term 'consumer' includes patients, the general public and consumer advocates. Consumer involvement refers to an active role in the research process, in contrast to the traditional use of consumers as the subjects of research. An investigation of consumer involvement in CAM research in the UK suggests that consumers are an underused resource and that many key players in the research enterprise have no experience of consumer involvement (Paterson 2004). Nevertheless, there are examples of successful consumer involvement at all stages of the research process, including the commissioning of research, protocol development and design, data collection and data analysis and the review and dissemination of outcomes. There are different degrees of consumer involvement, all of which can be useful. Consumers may lead the research process, may collaborate with researchers throughout a project or may be consulted by them regarding specific issues. Consumers can become enthusiastic and resourceful members of research teams and they can be useful and powerful allies for marginalised disciplines such as CAM.

In this chapter I explore what is meant by the concept of consumer involvement and then discuss some of the reasons why it is important to the research community. I then move on to illustrate how such ideas are being translated into practice and describe the experiences of CAM researchers and consumers in many different settings. The chapter draws upon results from my own recent work on consumer involvement in the field of CAM, as well as the work of others, to consider both the benefits and the problems of consumer involvement and how it can be extended and made more fruitful in the investigation of CAM.

What is consumer involvement?

Consumer involvement in research refers to their involvement in *doing* the research rather than involvement as research subjects. In this context, the word 'consumer' is used to denote a receiver, or potential receiver, of health care. In the UK, the NHS research and development programme uses the word 'consumer' to refer to people whose primary interest in health care is their own health, or that of their family, as past, current and potential patients, users of services or carers and people representing any of these groups through community organisations, networks or campaigning and self-help groups (Oliver et al. 2001). Alternative words, such as 'patient', 'service user', 'lay representative' and 'client' each have their protagonists and critics. The term 'consumer' has been criticised as only applicable to a market-orientated view of health care; the word 'patient' is disliked because of its overtones of sickness and disempowerment and the word 'user' is often associated with substance misuse (Boote et al. 2002). While acknowledging the different perceptions and arguments regarding these various terms, I do not wish to revisit this already well-versed area of debate. In this chapter I use these words interchangeably to encompass actual and potential recipients of health care, their families, non-professional carers and advocates.

In the context of consumers' roles in research, the term 'involvement' can also have a spectrum of meanings or levels. One useful framework describes three levels of consumer involvement: *user control, user collaboration* and *user consultation* (Hanley et al. 2003). User control is where consumers design, undertake and disseminate the results of a research project; user collaboration involves an active ongoing and reciprocal partnership of consumers and researchers in the research process; and user consultation refers to consumers being consulted by researchers, without necessarily implying reciprocity and shared power in decision-making. While this categorisation helps us to recognise the diversity and potential of these relationships, the boundary between collaboration and consultation is often difficult to define in practice (Telford et al. 2002). In addition to these direct methods of involvement, lay perspectives can be identified by reading lay publications and studies of people's views (Entwistle et al. 1998).

Why promote consumer involvement?

The two main reasons given for promoting the involvement of consumers in research are that it is morally correct and that it will improve the quality of the research. Morally, the argument is that in a democracy with a publicly funded health service the public have a right to influence how research funds are allocated and how research is done. This view is based on an understanding that different research benefits different people, and that health professionals and academic researchers are inevitably driven by their own professional and academic interests. CAM practitioners and researchers are no exception to this rule. In the UK, consumer involvement and 'consultation' has become politically sanctioned and the Department of Health (DoH) has provided clear expectations and guidance (DoH 2001) and an on-line source of free information and advice (INVOLVE at <http://www.invo.org.uk>). However, governments also have their own agendas and there is a danger that a narrow political focus on consumer involvement without the resources and time to make involvement meaningful can be used to legitimise political decisions.

The expectation that lay participation will improve the quality of the research rests, most broadly, on the recognition that there is a fundamental difference between the concepts of disease (a physiologic and clinical abnormality) and illness (the subjective experience of an individual). Consumers are expert in their illness and therefore 'when consumers' perspectives on illness are combined with clinicians' interests in disease, a synergistic relationship can exist and new insights can be gained to improve the condition of the consumer' (DoH 2001: 218). Again, CAM practitioners are not exempt from these circumstances. Even though CAM practitioners have a holistic approach that may include much of the patient's perspective, they still have their own therapeutic theory base that influences the way they make sense of that experience.

As a means of summarising the potential benefits of consumer involvement in research, we can follow the lead of Boote et al. (2002) who highlight that consumer involvement:

> ensures that issues which are important to consumers, and therefore to health services as a whole, are identified and prioritised; it ensured that money and resources are not wasted on research of little value; and it encourages consumers to push for outcomes that may have greater relevance than those considered by professionals. Consumers can also be instrumental in recruiting their peers to research projects, can help to access more marginalized members of society, and can disseminate research information to their peers.
>
> (Boote et al. 2002: 220)

Later in this chapter I will explore what evidence there is that such potential benefits exist in practice, especially in CAM research. First, I outline how CAM researchers and consumers are finding ways of working together and explore how consumer involvement is actually being done.

How is consumer involvement being done?

Investigations into the extent and manner of consumer involvement in health research in the UK to date includes a study of one NHS region (Telford et al.

2002), a review of involvement in clinical trials (Hanley et al. 2001), a study of the NHS Health Technology Assessment Programme (Oliver et al. 2001), an investigation of training provision and experiences (Lockey et al. 2004), and my own investigation of CAM research (Paterson 2003). All of these studies include the views of researchers but only the last three include interviews with consumers. In view of the considerable overlap in the findings of these studies, this chapter draws upon the CAM investigation in detail, and I refer to the other studies to embellish points as and when appropriate. I now provide an overview of my research into consumer involvement in CAM.

Consumer involvement in CAM research: findings from a contemporary study

The consumer involvement in CAM research study (CICAM), carried out in 2002–3, aimed to learn about consumer involvement in complementary medicine research from those with experience of practice in this area. A literature search was combined with written and oral responses from key people and organisations in the UK. The method and literature review is described in more detail elsewhere (Paterson 2003).

Literature review

Despite an extensive literature search, only six relevant papers and reports were identified. These were one workshop report, two reports from the Mental Health Foundation (MHF), one investigation into research priorities, one qualitative study and one policy document. This paucity of published material is reflected in the content of the first paper, an editorial that reports on a workshop on consumer involvement in CAM research (White and Barr 2001). Whilst the editorial is of general interest, none of the workshop participants had any direct experience of projects involving consumers.

The two reports from the MHF relate to a user-led project conducted by the foundation (MHF 1997), in which the activities, treatments and/or therapies deemed helpful by people with a range of different mental-health problems were explored. The project's focus included medication, electro convulsive therapy, 'talking treatments' (counselling and psychotherapy), alternative and complementary therapies, hobbies and leisure activities and religious and spiritual beliefs. The results are reported and discussed in some detail and the perspective of mental-health users and survivors is maintained throughout the report.

The MHF published a second report entitled *Healing Minds* drawing upon the results of the first report and discussing current research policy and practice concerning the use of complementary and alternative therapies for a wide range of mental-health problems (Wallcraft 1998). The author also draws on other user-led surveys, evaluations and personal accounts, but these are all unpublished, or published as newspaper articles or consumer-organisation newsletters (and consequently were not identified by my more academic search strategy). This second MHF report makes ten recommendations, several of which relate to user involvement in research, such as 'no existing therapy should be considered as having been proven to be safe and effective in mental health if service users and/or their organisations have not been involved in the design of the outcome measures used' (Wallcraft 1998: 71).

The fourth paper in the CICAM review, an investigation into research priorities for the treatment of osteoarthritis, reports on a mismatch between the agendas of the research community and the research consumer (Tallon et al. 2000). A review of the research literature identified a massive concentration of research into drug and surgical treatments, but when patients with osteoarthritis of the knee were consulted they favoured conservative treatment, such as physiotherapy and complementary medicine, and wanted more research on education and self-help. Professional groups also perceived oral drugs as over-researched and wanted high-quality evidence for all types of interventions. The authors conclude that the research agenda needs to be broadened if it is to reflect current treatment patterns and consumer views. The last two papers in the CICAM review are from the USA. An in-depth qualitative study of both users and practitioners of Chinese medicine describes how patients were involved in piloting an interview schedule and a questionnaire and how these tools had been revised several times during this piloting process (Ma 1999), and a report on a public-consultation exercise exploring how public-policy changes might be used to help disseminate CAM research findings (Fritts 2000).

The CICAM literature review suggests that either there is little consumer involvement in CAM research or such research is not often being written about in peer-reviewed papers. A similar conclusion was drawn by Telford et al. (2002) with respect to consumer involvement in all types of research. However, the consumer-led investigation by Wallcraft (1998), described above, found some material that was published as newspaper articles, consumer-organisation newsletters and personal accounts. This raises issues about what type of knowledge is valued and listed in academia and the difficulties of accessing lay and non-academic material.

Key people and organisations

The second part of the CICAM study consulted key people and organisations in the following categories: consumer groups and charities, researchers known to be involved in research into complementary medicine or into consumer involvement, professional complementary medicine organisations and other relevant organisations. Fifty-nine people or organisations were contacted and forty-three people (73 per cent) responded. Contact and responses were by telephone, email or letter and included both people who had, and those who had not had, experience of consumer involvement. Eighteen people were interviewed, which included everyone with any personal experience of consumer involvement.

Findings

Extent of consumer involvement

The first round of email responses included five university departments that were renowned for research into complementary medicine with four identifying they had no experience of involving consumers in research. One of these university departments had facilitated a workshop on the subject where attendees had been enthusiastic but had no experience to share. Meanwhile, the head of another university department had some experience of trying to involve consumers but without success:

> All sorts of different funding bodies want you to get 'the patient's view-point' but it's actually almost impossible to get an expert patient ... I haven't really been able to get hold of anybody appropriate, even from a patient-based charity ... It's all very well thinking of involving patients, how do you actually go about it?
>
> (Head of Research Unit)

Most of the other researchers contacted in the CICAM study had not considered involving consumers in their own research. The professional complementary medicine organisations and the consumer organisations/charities did not all respond to the inquiry, but most of those that did reply had no experience to report. An interviewee from the Arthritis Research Campaign said he was 'feeling his way' and suggested that most people were unsure how to take consumer involvement forward, how to get the right sort of person involved and how to avoid consumers being overwhelmed with the medical and professional jargon. This level of consumer involvement in CAM research mirrors findings in other types of research. For example, less than a third of NHS trusts in one region were involving consumers in research and only twenty-three of sixty-two clinical trial coordinating centres had done so between 1990 and 1998.

It is against this backdrop of a low level of consumer involvement that consumers and researchers who did have experience to share were interviewed. These twelve interviews spanned all three levels of involvement (user control, user collaboration and user consultation) as identified by Hanley et al. (2003). These categories will here be used to describe the scope and manner of involvement identified, prior to describing the perceived benefits and problems of such involvement in more detail and how the process might be improved.

User-led research

The CICAM investigation included four user-led research organisations or projects and a wide range of experiences. The Alzheimer's Society is a national consumer organisation that involves its members in all stages of the research process, and one consumer (of a group of three) and one researcher involved in their trial of gingko biloba in dementia were interviewed. They noted that in nominating and prioritising research areas and projects, consumers gave high priority and support to CAM. Consumer leadership in nominating, prioritising, selecting and monitoring this particular trial was described as a positive experience for both consumer and researcher. The consumer found her role interesting and enjoyed the informal training opportunities, and the researcher especially valued the transparent process and the consumer input into recruitment procedures.

The Parkinson's Disease Society (PDS) provided an example of user-led research on a much smaller scale, with a local branch using national PDS funding to provide and evaluate massage therapy for some of their members. Researchers were recruited to lead the study design and analysis, and the consumers managed the budget, took part in data collection and discussed the results. Moreover, the consumer knowledge of the effects and limitations of Parkinson's disease were crucial to designing a feasible study. The Herpes Viruses Association (HVA), a smaller national organisation, provided a different model of involvement based on 'in-house' trials of over-the-counter or Internet-marketed products. Members participated in these trials and used the results for their own self-management as well as publishing results in the association's newsletter and elsewhere. Although the HVA newsletter is regularly used by research units to recruit patients to trials and members have also been involved in one-off consultation requests by outside researchers, participants perceived research as often elitist and dominated by pharmaceutical company funding. The fourth interview concerning user-led research was with a consumer who had made many unsuccessful attempts to fund research into treating asthma with speleotherapy. Despite setting up the Speleotherapy Foundation and leading a Cochrane review, this interviewee described the difficulties faced by consumers who wish to initiate research.

Collaboration: an active ongoing partnership of consumers in the research process

Four people provided several examples of collaborative research. A consumer representative on the advisory board of the Complementary Medicine Field of the Cochrane Collaboration described her experience of commenting on Cochrane systematic reviews, and her knowledge of the Cochrane consumer network (see <http://www.cochrane.org/consumers>; for discussion of systematic reviews and the Cochrane Collaboration relating to CAM, see

Manheimer and Ezzo, Chapter 4). Her systematic review work involves commenting on the language used in a review, the need to avoid abbreviations and checking that there is a section exploring unintended effects. She was also part of a research team running a randomised trial of acupuncture for headache where her contribution on the debate around financial incentives for participants had been especially useful. This interviewee was in favour of funding bodies insisting on consumer involvement, had plenty of suggestions about 'finding' suitable people and thought that researchers should not become immobilised by seeking the perfect consumer representative.

A second interviewee described how, as chair of the local BackCare charity, he had been recruited to join a research team running a large-scale trial of acupuncture for back pain. During the interview he drew on not only his own experiences and views, but those of many other patients too and he saw his involvement in research as an opportunity to provide feedback on this experience and to fulfil a useful role. This interviewee found that he was able to contribute the patient's perspective, especially in designing questionnaires, but would have liked a clearer statement of the roles of all research-team members. He also highlighted the need to take into account the illness-related limitations of many consumers and the need to pay expenses and expressed some dismay at the overall cost of the research trial. The researchers on the same trial had involved this consumer as an essential requirement from their funder but found it a beneficial experience and went on to consult consumers in a subsequent trial of acupuncture for depression. This time the researchers consulted consumers early in the planning stage and the mental-health charity Mind organised a day when a group of eight consumers met to discuss their experience of depression and the design of the study. Not only did this help clarify concerns about the control group, but Mind also offered to organise and fund counselling for trial participants should they require it. The junior researcher on this project found the experience very supportive and expressed a desire to invite individuals from the group to join the research team if and when funding was secured.

Consultation: where consumers are consulted with no sharing of power in decision-making

At a Macmillan cancer support centre, consumer involvement was integral to most activities, such as publishing information, but only recently had focus groups been used to discuss specific aspects of research design. Useful insights from such groups, such as how a personalised appointment for aromatherapy is a stronger motivation to attend than the invitation to participate in a group relaxation session, have led to increasing consultation. Another project that arose from consumer demand and has community members on its steering group was an integrated health-care project where the researcher had consulted widely about her information sheet, with the result that it used large type and pictures, included more information rather than less and was available on tape. However, she was not aware that ethics committees would allow patient involvement in other areas such as research design.

The final interviewees were the director, and patient adviser, of the Institute for Musculoskeletal Research and Clinical Implementation. The patient adviser was recovering from many years of severe back pain and disability, and she hoped that research would prevent others having similar experiences to her own. She had previously set up a support group for people in chronic pain and both this, and her research involvement, had enabled her to turn her bad experiences into something positive and useful. Her husband, who accompanied her as her carer, also became involved and offers a separate carer perspective. Their current involvement consists of spending over a day at the research centre several times a year, and since travel and overnight expenses are paid they are able to enjoy this trip away from home. Meanwhile, the researcher had found the input of the patient and her husband invaluable, especially their practical advice about experiencing the diagnostic and treatment procedures. However, the researcher explained how he had also experienced other consumer involvement in multidisciplinary advisory panels where roles had been unclear and consumers had not been able to contribute usefully. Despite his enthusiasm for consumer involvement on specific projects, he was unsure as to whether lay consumer involvement was appropriate for either setting research priorities or for certain types of research such as surveys of professional behaviour. In a project that was developing guidelines for clinicians, he saw those clinicians as consumers and he emphasised that because his research centre was outside the orthodox research community he had to work hard at collaboration across all groups and consumers. In this respect, consumer involvement was the key to ensuring maximum implementation of research findings.

What are the benefits and the costs of consumer involvement?

The UK DoH research governance framework includes consideration of consumer involvement at three stages of research: in protocol development, in the execution of research and development (the doing of research) and in the review and dissemination of outcomes. This is a useful framework to explore the CICAM findings regarding the benefits and costs of consumer involvement.

The CICAM project suggests that priority-setting and protocol development is the area that experiences least consumer involvement and where researchers express the most doubts about such involvement. However, where consumer involvement has taken place at this level (by means of consumer leadership as in the Alzheimer's Society programme, or by increasing researcher confidence, as in the case of the acupuncture research trials in back pain and depression), the process appears to be mutually beneficial. Consumer involvement can add enthusiasm and energy to the team, ensure that the research is grounded in real-life problems, foresee problems with recruitment and retention of patients, help in the choice of outcome measures, tackle ethical problems, offer practical and personal support to researchers and assist with funding. The costs are those involved in setting up and using a consumer network or small group and integrating this with the work of the research team. These costs may occur before any research funding is secured, and in the examples in this study they were mainly borne by the consumers and their organisations. Other 'costs', particularly for researchers, relate to giving up some power and control. That this issue did not feature much in this investigation may be because of the focus on exploring actual experiences.

The CICAM study shows that consumer participation in the 'doing' of research is more widespread. Indeed, it took place across the whole spectrum of involvement, from long-term collaborations to brief task-orientated consultation. The patient perspective appears particularly useful for producing accessible and appropriate written information for participants and for avoiding recruitment problems. Research led by consumer organisations involved recruiting enthusiastic participants directly from their membership, and collaborations with consumers allowed access to members via internal newsletters. Not only did the consumer perspective help develop a more effective 'sales pitch' for recruitment, but it also helped research participants through minimising the distress and disruption of the research procedures and follow-up. Costs of participation in this area depend on the level of involvement and are sometimes, but not always, paid from the research-project funds. Short-term consultation usually requires a meeting place, travel expenses and, preferably, a good meal. Longer-term collaborations were found to require more organisational input and more time commitment.

The area of reviewing and disseminating research results was one where individual researchers often took their 'first steps' towards consumer involvement. Trial participants gave useful feedback and insights into how a design had worked out in practice and often helped to interpret the meanings behind numerical results. Involving consumers in multidisciplinary teams or advisory boards, with a view to maximising the implementation of the research findings, may be especially important for marginalised areas of research such as complementary medicine. The dissemination of research findings in lay publications, in a form that the general public can understand, helps consumers to make their own treatment decisions and to refer to a research base when negotiating for appropriate NHS health care. The Cochrane Consumer Network (see <http://www.cochrane.org/consumers>) is evidence of the scope for consumer involvement in reviews of evidence.

Consumers in the CICAM study describe several ways in which they have benefited from participation in research. Several people explained how involvement in research allowed them to turn a bad experience of illness into a positive contribution to the common good. People talked about the self-encouragement that involvement in research provided and a sense that 'something was being done'. Participants also expressed their interest in engaging in the process and the new social opportunities that such involvement afforded them. Some negative consequences of research involvement described by the participants included frustration at being unable to influence the medical research establishment, being restricted by financial and health considerations and the surprise and anxiety at the money that research consumes.

Objections to consumer involvement

In their review of consumer involvement in health research, Boote et al. (2002) describe seven areas of objection that have been voiced by clinicians and researchers. Although some of these were voiced by the CAM researchers and practitioners that I interviewed in the CICAM study, it is likely that the focus on actual experience of involvement resulted in an under-representation of negative views. Nevertheless, these potential objections are worth considering in more detail and, despite the limitations of the CICAM sample, I here examine each from the perspective of the consumers that were interviewed.

Representativeness

A common concern among researchers is that the consumer who takes part in research will not be representative of all consumers in the research area. It has been suggested that consulting a number of consumers, or consulting in different ways, such as with individuals and focus groups, may help to overcome this problem. The CICAM data suggests that once CAM researchers become involved with consumers this particular concern tends to fade and the individual contributions that one or more consumers bring to the project are valued in their own right. The consumers I spoke to or heard about all had connections, often strong ones, with a consumer organisation, health charity or support group. Although these people draw on knowledge and experience gathered through their organisational link and sometimes use their organisations for support, none of them refer to themselves as patient representatives or advocates. Rather, they provide 'a consumer perspective' based on being a patient, or carer, or lay consumer of health-care information. This focus on a consumer perspective, rather than a consumer representative, has been advocated by others (Hanley et al. 2003).

Quality

Many professionals are concerned that the contribution of lay people may be severely limited by a lack of understanding of the complexities and rigour of research. In addition, these commentators also suggest that other skills and qualities are required by research participants such as organisational and computer skills and the ability to work in teams. However, as the CICAM study illustrates, the Alzheimer Society has demonstrated that, with appropriate training, consumers can contribute to all stages of the research enterprise. The researcher in the Alzheimer Society CAM trial found consumer input useful and encouraging as well as aiding the transparency of the research process. What is clear from the accounts of these researchers is that consumer input is in addition to, not instead of, orthodox science. The consumer in the acupuncture and back-pain trial explained how he discovered that everyone in the research enterprise was specialising in their own areas of expertise and that his contribution came from his knowledge of the experience of living with back pain. He found that his ignorance of statistics, for example, was no greater than the statistician's ignorance of the patient experience.

A variety of models for research skills training are available (INVOLVE at <http://www.invo.org.uk/training.asp>), and training programmes for consumer involvement in service planning can be readily adapted for a research programme. The consumers interviewed in the CICAM study generally preferred one-on-one discussions with researchers when particular issues emerged to more formal training, in line with the suggestion of mentorship that emerged from the Health Technology Assessment pilot study. Others have made the point that training needs are not one-sided, and that researchers too may need to learn new skills and attitudes (Oliver 1999). However, an in-depth investigation of training provision and participants' experiences suggests that if training is participative and carefully targeted it can play a vital role in facilitating consumer involvement in research (Lockey et al. 2004). This investigation concludes that training is perceived as being most useful when it has a clear aim and purpose and is centred around specific research tasks and real research problems that draw upon the participants' experiences. Lockey et al. (2004) found that participants wanted to be involved in creating and developing ideas in which they could become absorbed and take some level of ownership, and that a key aspect of successful training was exchange and sharing between people, both trainers and participants. The research also found that training helped affirm the strength and value of service users' experiences and understanding of health conditions and services. Training was identified as having enormous value for participants' personal development and confidence and, almost without exception, led to actual involvement in research and a desire to do more. Lastly, Lockey et al. (2004) identified language as a significant challenge for those providing training, but effective training 'demystified' research, providing a base from which stakeholders could understand one another's language and purpose.

Bias

Researchers that view academia as developing knowledge in an impartial and objective fashion may be worried by the input of consumers whose contributions come from their own individual experience. While individual biases are inevitable amongst all members of the team, the power and depth of the individual lived experience is also the strength of the consumer perspective. In the CICAM study, both researchers and consumers agreed that it was an advantage to have consumers who had contacts with support groups or consumer organisations and who were therefore in a position to reflect on a variety of lay experiences. It was also highlighted as important that all members of the research team acknowledge that there are a wide variety of experiences and perspectives, all of which should be respected.

Influence

Consumer involvement in research may diminish the researcher's power and control over the course of the project. Not too surprisingly, such a change in power does face objections from some researchers despite the potential benefits to consumers. In the user-led Alzheimer's disease trial identified in the CICAM study there had been changes to the original design including long and difficult discussions over inclusion criteria, but the researcher did not feel disempowered by the process. Similarly, the design of the acupuncture and depression trial was substantially changed by the consumer focus group, but the junior researcher experienced the process as very supportive.

Consumer expectations

Some researchers are anxious that consumers may have unrealistic expectations about what an individual research project can achieve and that, consequently, they will be dissatisfied with research plans or results. In the CICAM research, this concern was expressed, for example, by a researcher running a clinical trial who suggested that a clearer remit for consumers would be helpful, and both researchers and consumers emphasised the importance of consumers knowing what is expected of them and of having tasks clearly set. However, it was also clear that consumers had useful contributions to make in areas that were not initially prioritised as relevant.

Researchers did not always know where the consumer's perspective was appropriate and helpful, such as in making ethical decisions, in dissemination of findings and in planning further work. The ability of consumers to expand their remit depends on gaining confidence over time in a research environment that is consumer-friendly. Consumer expectations may pose a challenge to researchers in other ways too, as exemplified by a consumer in the CICAM study who was dismayed at the cost of the trial and questioned whether it was the best use of NHS money.

Increased cost and length of research

It is inevitable that consumer involvement costs both time and money, and the importance of this practical barrier should not be underestimated (Redfern et al. 2004, Belam et al. 2005). Recouping these costs within the research grant can be difficult, but should be given priority in developing funding applications. The value of consumers as advocates and their role in submitting successful funding bids were noted by the clinical-trial researchers surveyed by Hanley et al. (2001). Clear guidelines are now available about the payment of consumer representatives (<http://www.invo.org.uk/Publication_Guidelines.asp>), and consumer remuneration is usually much less than those of many other members of the research team. Furthermore, consumer payment can actually bring some monetary advantages, such as the considerable savings made by improved recruitment and completion rates. Some researchers have also been able to involve the same consumers on several occasions, a process that builds fruitful relationships and experience as well as being cost-effective on training and mentoring. This design feature could be developed further by NHS trusts or academic departments facilitating more centralised resources.

Overlapping roles

The argument that health practitioners are also consumers and can therefore represent consumer issues may be one of particular cognisance to CAM practitioners who value their holistic approach and egalitarian relationships. That patients have different perspectives and priorities regarding their health and treatment options than their conventional practitioners is well documented (KellyPowell 1997, Edwards et al. 2002, Lapsley and Groves 2004), and there are also numerous examples of how attending to lay perspectives has caused biomedical researchers to review their methods (O'Brien, 1993, Bradburn et al. 1995). Whether such differences occur between patients and CAM practitioners have not, to my knowledge, been investigated, but the enthusiasm for involving consumers exhibited by some of the CAM practitioners interviewed in the CICAM study suggests that direct consumer involvement does add new and valuable information. For example, the chiropractor who leads the Institute for Musculoskeletal Research and Clinical

Implementation found his patient adviser so useful that he funded hotel and subsistence expenses for her and her carer several times a year.

How can consumer involvement in CAM be increased and more effective?

The list of potential problems associated with consumer involvement in research as outlined above has originated from the views of researchers and health professionals, rather than those of consumers. Analysis of the interviews with consumers in the CICAM study suggests that there are several other aspects that need to be attended to in order to make their involvement more fruitful and meaningful. Bastian (1995) suggests that in addition to attending to expectations and goals, as described above, two more elements need to be attended to: the characteristics of the people themselves and the environment in which they work.

Most of the consumers interviewed in the CICAM study had a personal, often extensive and distressing, experience of illness and they all had connections with a consumer organisation, health charity or support group. Some of them used this group as a source of support. Two further attributes were frequently mentioned: having recovered or learnt to live with illness and being involved in helping others.

More generally, people usually needed to be confident enough to work in a group and ask questions, although sometimes involvement was via written or e-mailed communication, or in a one-to-one situation. Consumers were contacted by researchers in many different ways including direct approaches to consumer organisations or support groups, advertisements in the organisation's newsletter, requests to attend a group meeting to discuss the research or even asking if a special focus group could be formed for the purpose. Other suggestions were advertising in national consumer health magazines, advertising in surgeries and hospitals or asking health-care professionals to broach and discuss the topic with suitable patients. Initially, consulting a group of consumers and selecting a smaller number from this group for more long-term collaboration is one strategy for finding consumers who may enjoy contributing positively in a research team environment. It is notable that consumers who wanted to find researchers to work with were, in the CICAM investigation, only successful when they had access to funding or funding opportunities.

The CICAM study shows that consumers are involved in CAM research by means of group meetings, postal and email correspondence, one-to-one discussions and focus groups; such rich experiences gave rise to many suggestions about how to make the research environment more consumer-friendly. Most important perhaps, is the extent to which researchers and doctors appear able to learn to explain and discuss issues in accessible and jargon-free language. The issue of language is also highlighted by consumers in the study by Oliver et al. (2001) who found difficulty with management and committee terminology as well as medical terminology such as 'speaking through the chair', 'secondary publications', trajectory' and 'diffusion curve'.

In the CICAM study, consumers who were involved in research team meetings often needed an opportunity to reflect and respond after as well as during the meeting. Consumers explained their need to know not only their own roles and tasks, but also the perspectives of the others involved, and they expressed their appreciation at the opportunity to share experiences and build relationships. There were several examples of researchers, as well as consumers, appreciating this building of mutual respect and a supportive environment. Several consumers were lone lay voices in research groups, but they did not all see this as a problem. Indeed, many consumers expressed some anxiety about being asked to work with other consumers who they might find intimidating or difficult. More problematic was being asked to join a research team that was already well established, and when this is inevitable, time needs to be put aside for full introductions including clarity about each person's role within the team. The research environment also needs to take into account the difficulties experienced by consumers who are living with a chronic health problem, such as difficulties with access, travel and finances.

Many of these issues have been raised by consumers before (Bastian 1994), and evidence suggests that when they are ignored it is difficult for consumers to influence research agendas. While consumer-led research largely circumvents these barriers, it may face particular problems accessing research funding and facilities.

Conclusion

As this chapter illustrates, the consumer perspective is important and useful at all stages of the research process. The literature provides examples of successful consumer involvement in commissioning research, protocol development, all aspects of carrying out research and in the review and dissemination of outcomes. Consumers may lead the research process, collaborate with researchers throughout a project or be consulted by them on specific issues. There is evidence that participation at all of these levels of research can be useful and fulfilling.

Consumers are an underused resource in CAM research and many key players in the CAM research field appear to have no experience of consumer involvement. The academic research departments investigated in the CICAM study were aware of the concept but had difficulty putting it into practice, and some individual researchers, particularly practitioner researchers, appeared to be considering the idea for the first time. Even organisations committed to consumer involvement in service provision found it difficult to conceive of collaboration at all stages of research. Where involvement had taken place, this was generally because funding bodies demanded it or because consumers had taken the lead in research. Those committed to multidisciplinary work were also playing a lead role, viewing lay representatives as just one more perspective to take on board.

Nevertheless, there are some inspiring examples of consumer involvement in CAM research and much can be learnt from other people's experiences. Most consumers who participated in the CICAM study were connected to a consumer organisation or support group, but perceived themselves as offering an individual consumer perspective. The ability of consumers to contribute to CAM research appears to depend on a consumer-friendly research environment and clear roles and tasks. As consumers gain confidence they are able to widen their areas of involvement.

Although most CAM researchers investigated began involving consumers in order to comply with the requirements of funding bodies, the experience of working together usually led to an appreciation of the value of the consumer perspective. In this sense, researchers were identified as moving from a position of compliance to one of enthusiasm for consumer involvement. The experience of collaboration led several people to suggest that CAM should be at the forefront of involving consumers, because consumers can be useful and powerful allies for marginalised disciplines such as complementary medicine. This viewpoint was supported by published reports of the views of people with osteoarthritis and mental-health problems.

From the research experiences identified in the CICAM study there appears to be more than one productive model for researcher and consumer-research involvement. However, mutual respect and clear communication between individuals and groups does appear to be a key component of any successful collaboration. Consumer involvement is a challenge facing CAM researchers, and all who contribute and aid CAM research. While the barriers to consumer involvement within this field appear to be similar to those identified in other research areas, the need for involvement and the potential benefits for both individual researchers and the field as a whole may prove to be highly significant for a marginalised discipline such as CAM.

References

Bastian, H. (1995) *The Power of Sharing Knowledge*, Oxford: UK Cochrane Centre.

Belam, J., Harris, G., Kernick, D. P., Kline, F., Lindley, K., McWatt, J., Mitchell, A. and Reinhold, D. (2005) 'A qualitative study of migraine involving patient researchers', *British Journal of General Practice*, 55 (511): 87–93.

Boote, J., Telford, R. and Cooper, C. L. (2002) 'Consumer involvement in health research: a review and research agenda', *Health Policy*, 61 (2): 213–36.

Bradburn, J., Maher, J., Adewuyidalton, R., Grunfeld, E., Lancaster, T. and Mant, D. (1995) 'Developing clinical trial protocols: the use of patient focus groups', *Psycho-oncology*, 4 (2): 107–12.

Department of Health (2001) 'Research Governance Framework for Health and Social Care'. Available at <http://www.dh.gov.uk/assetRoot/04/01/47/57/04014757.pdf>. (Accessed June 2005.)

Edwards, S. G. M., Playford, E. D., Hobart, J. C. and Thompson, A. J. (2002) 'Comparison of physician outcome measures and patients' perception of benefits of inpatient neurorehabilitation', *British Medical Journal*, 324 (7352): 1493.

Entwistle, V. A., Renfrew, M. J., Yearley, S., Forrester, J. and Lamont, T. (1998) 'Lay perspectives: advantages for health research', *British Medical Journal*, 316 (7129): 463–6.

Fritts, M. (2000) 'News item about the White House Commission on CAM policy', *Journal of the National Cancer Institute*, 92 (24): 1975–6.

Hanley, B., Truesdale, A., King, A., Elbourne, D. and Chalmers, I. (2001) 'Involving consumers in designing, conducting, and interpreting randomised controlled trials; questionnaire survey', *British Medical Journal*, 322 (7285): 519–23.

Hanley, B., Bradburn, J., Gorin, S., Barnes, M., Evans, C. and Goodare, H. (2003) 'Involving the Public in NHS, Public Health and Social Care Research: Briefing notes for Researchers'. Available online at <http://www.invo.org.uk>.

KellyPowell, M. L. (1997) 'Personalizing choices: patients experiences with making treatment decisions', *Research in Nursing and Health*, 20 (3): 219–27.

Lapsley, P. and Groves, T. (2004) 'The patient's journey: travelling through life with a chronic illness. A new BMJ series to deepen doctors' understanding', *British Medical Journal*, 329 (7466): 582–3.

Lockey, R., Sitzia, J., Gillingham, T., Millyard, J., Miller, C. and Ahmend, S. (2004) 'Training for service user involvement in health and social care research: a study of training provision and participants' experiences (the TRUE project)'. Available online at <http://www.invo.org.uk/Training.asp>. (Accessed 23 July 2005.)

Ma, G. X. (1999) 'Between two worlds: the use of traditional and western health services by Chinese immigrants', *Journal of Community Health*, 24 (6): 421–37.

Mental Health Foundation (1997) *Knowing Our Own Minds*, London: Mental Health Foundation.

O'Brien, K. (1993) 'Using focus groups to develop health surveys: an example from research on social relationships and AIDS-preventive behaviour', *Health Education Quarterly*, 20 (3): 361–72.

Oliver, S. (1999) 'Has involving consumers (patients) in research made any difference to what is researched and how?', *Journal of Health Services Research and Policy*, 4 (2): 127–8.

Oliver, S., Milne, R., Bradburn, J., Buchanan, P., Kerridge, L. and Walley, T. (2001) 'Involving consumers in a needs-led research programme: a pilot project', *Health Expectations*, 4 (1): 18–28.

Paterson, C. (2003) 'Consumer involvement in research into complementary and alternative therapies'. Available online at <http://www.hsrc.ac.uk/Current_research/research_programmes/research_link.htm>. (Accessed 23 July 2005.)

—— (2004) 'Take small steps to go a long way' consumer involvement in research into complementary and alternative therapies', *Complementary Therapies in Nursing and Midwifery*, 10 (3): 150–61.

Redfern, J., McKevitt, C. and Wolfe, C. (2004) 'The MRC Framework for developing and evaluating complex interventions: putting the theory into practice', *Journal of Epidemiology and Community Health*, 58 (Supplement II): A3.

Tallon, D., Chard, J. and Dieppe, P. (2000) 'Relation between agendas of the research community and the research consumer', *Lancet*, 355 (9220): 2037–40.

Telford, R., Beverley, C. A., Cooper, C. L. and Boote, J. D. (2002) 'Consumer involvement in health research: fact or fiction?', *British Journal of Clinical Governance*, 7 (2): 92–103.

Wallcraft, J. (1998) *Healing Minds: A Report on Current Research, Policy and Practice Concerning the Use of Complementary and Alternative Therapies for a Wide Range of Mental Health Problems*, London: Mental Health Foundation.

White, A. and Barr, G. (2001) 'Consumer involvement in CAM research', *Complementary Therapies in Medicine*, 9 (4): 205–6.

Index